101 QUESTIONS AND ANSWERS ABOUT

Carpal Tunnel Syndrome

101 QUESTIONS AND ANSWERS ABOUT

Carpal Tunnel Syndrome

What It Is, How to Prevent It, and Where to Turn for Treatment

Steven J. McCabe, M.D.

Contemporary Books

Chicago New York San Francisco Lisbon London Madrid Mexico City
Milan New Delhi San Juan Seoul Singapore Sydney Toronto

The intent of this book is to provide accurate medical information about a common condition; however, no book can replace careful evaluation and treatment by your doctor. If you are experiencing a hand problem, this book can provide information to help you to participate, along with your doctor, in your own care. This is the appropriate and beneficial use for what you will learn from this book.

Library of Congress Cataloging-in-Publication Data
McCabe, Steven J.
    101 questions and answers about carpal tunnel syndrome / Steven J. McCabe.
      p. cm.
    Includes bibliographical references and index.
    ISBN 0-7373-0592-4
    1. Carpal tunnel syndrome—Popular works. I. Title: One hundred one questions and answers about carpal tunnel syndrome.

    RC422.C26 M38 2002
    616.8′7—dc21

                                  2001055964

Contemporary Books

*A Division of The **McGraw·Hill** Companies*

1 2 3 4 5 6 7 8 9 10   AGM/AGM 1 10 9 8 7 6 5 4 3 2

ISBN 0-7373-0592-4

This book was set in Minion by Robert S. Tinnon Design
Printed and bound by Quebecor Martinsburg

Interior design by Robert S. Tinnon
Interior illustrations by Elaine Bammerlin, M.A., C.M.I.

McGraw-Hill books are available at special quantity discounts to use as premiums and sales promotions, or for use in corporate training programs. For more information, please write to the Director of Special Sales, Professional Publishing, McGraw-Hill, Two Penn Plaza, New York, NY 10121-2298. Or contact your local bookstore.

This book is printed on acid-free paper.

This book is dedicated to my parents,
who deserve the credit for getting me
through medical school when I was at an age
when I really didn't have the wisdom or foresight
to know the importance of my own education.
They gave me genetic ability, a stable home,
the drive to withstand the academic rigor,
and the financial support necessary to
put me in the position to allow
me to write this book.

Thank you.

Contents

PART THREE

History and Epidemiology: Carpal Tunnel Syndrome over Time and in Populations   31

PART FOUR
Hands at Work: Carpal Tunnel Syndrome, the Workplace, and the Repetitive Stress Injury Controversy   41

PART FIVE
Getting Help: How Doctors Diagnose and Treat Carpal Tunnel Syndrome   53

PART SIX
Surgical Solutions: Surgery for Carpal Tunnel Syndrome   77

PART SEVEN

Tradition and Innovation: The Benefits and Risks of Traditional and Endoscopic Surgery   95

Foreword

Carpal tunnel syndrome is a complex physical condition comprising complex medical, legal, and societal factors. Intense controversy about the cause, the treatment, and even the definition of carpal tunnel syndrome has enveloped the medical community. Research in this area has done as much to cloud as to clarify our understanding. It is no surprise that patients with pain and numbness in their hands encounter confusion, misinformation, and even discrimination as they attempt to seek treatment for these disabling symptoms. In *101 Questions and Answers About Carpal Tunnel Syndrome*, Steve McCabe, M.D., brings his unusual training and years of experience to the aid of patients with carpal tunnel syndrome.

Dr. McCabe is one of the best-known and most respected hand surgeons in the United States. His graduate training in biostatistics, epidemiology, and research design gives him an enhanced ability to critically evaluate the current literature in this area. He has taken this depth of understanding of carpal tunnel syndrome and has written a clear, concise, and accessible book that gives a balanced presentation of the controversies about this topic in a nonjudgmental fashion. The clear, everyday language and the question-and-answer format make this book readable; the absence of bias or preaching makes this book valuable. We do not know all the factors that cause carpal tunnel syndrome. We do not know all the factors that determine its severity or the disability it produces in individual patients. We do not know how to treat carpal tunnel syndrome in an optimal fashion for all patients. We do know, however, that only a rational, balanced approach to this problem will allow optimal treatment for each patient now and enable us to move forward with worthwhile research in the future. This book will help patients with carpal tunnel syndrome to become active participants in their own treatment and will serve to emphasize to physicians the therapeutic benefit of a tempered, humanistic approach to afflicted patients. Carpal tunnel syndrome is a real problem; this book is a step toward a real solution.

WILLIAM M. KUZON, JR., M.D., PH.D.
ASSOCIATE PROFESSOR
PLASTIC AND RECONSTRUCTIVE SURGERY
UNIVERSITY OF MICHIGAN

Preface

Carpal tunnel syndrome, though not life threatening, is one of the most common medical problems of our times. Although it was first identified and defined over a century ago, it has become controversial only in the past thirty years.

Carpal tunnel syndrome is also a "chameleon" that takes on a different appearance and coloration depending on who is looking at it. Surgeons see it as a pinched nerve to be fixed through a variety of treatments and surgical procedures. Some businesses see it as a threat to profitability; others, as offering the potential for huge profits in the growing areas of ergonomics and injury prevention. Government regulatory agencies see it as a cumulative trauma disorder to be prevented.

But if you're a patient with carpal tunnel syndrome, it's first and foremost a source of day-to-day suffering that can range from intermittent discomfort to crippling pain that wreaks havoc not just with your body but with every aspect of your daily life.

Carpal tunnel syndrome describes more than just the pinching of the median nerve in the wrist. It has become a kind of symbol that reflects certain societal values and tensions, so to some extent its identification, diagnosis, evaluation, and treatment are, like all diseases and the symptoms they cause, molded not just by the condition itself but also by where we are as a society.

This book offers a great deal of information from the perspective of the hand surgeon using the traditional medical approach for carpal tunnel syndrome. This approach is grounded in medical science and has helped many patients over a long period of time. In short, I believe carpal tunnel syndrome itself is a simple medical condition based on very clear anatomical and physiological factors, but when it involves individuals it becomes complex. Although I take a "mechanical" approach to this condition, I do not ignore the controversy, and later in the book I discuss some of the features of the current debate over repetitive strain injury.

I've written this book to give health consumers the most accurate, detailed, and up-to-date information available about carpal tunnel syndrome in a format that's easy to read and understand. The development of the Internet has resulted in an explosion of health-care information that's now available to any consumer with a computer and a modem. Because carpal tunnel syndrome is so prevalent, many Web sites focus on it. Personally, I have been disappointed by the quality of much of that information. Too many of the descriptions are superficial or inaccurate, or obviously geared mainly at selling a product.

I've tried to give you, the reader, as much information as possible so you can take charge of your own life and well-being, but I encourage you not to delay in seeking medical advice if you're experiencing any troubling symptoms. Occasionally, serious conditions arise, and this book is not intended to be a substitute for professional medical advice.

It is my hope that these 101 questions and answers will be helpful for a wide range of readers: for those of you experiencing hand numbness and those worried that carpal tunnel syndrome may be the cause; for those who are weighing whether to seek treatment of various kinds; for those who are considering surgery or have already undergone it; and finally, for those who, like myself, are fascinated by one of the most complex and exasperating medical conditions of our postmodern era.

Acknowledgments

Through the years, I've learned a great deal from my patients, and I thank them for that. The study of medicine and surgery provides a framework of knowledge, but reading from a book or journal lacks texture and context. The experiences gained from taking care of people with problems add the details. My patients have actually written this book by asking questions about carpal tunnel syndrome. I've merely added answers and passed along their questions so that people with an interest can learn about their hands.

As surgeons, we would be nothing without our teachers. Seldom does a student surpass his or her teacher; at best, we can absorb some of the qualities, abilities, and skills of those we admire and respect. My colleagues, Harold E. Kleinert, M.D., James F. Murray, M.D., Robert M. McFarlane, M.D., and Joseph E. Kutz, M.D., have all reinforced my interest and ability in hand surgery, not as much as they would have liked to, I'm sure, but to a serviceable degree. I'll never attain their level of skill and ability, but I've tried to take something from each and do my best with it.

Hand surgery is a career, a research endeavor, a curriculum, and a hobby. For most hand surgeons, it is totally preoccupying. Without the support of an understanding wife and family, none of us would find it possible to write, teach, or do research. Thank you, Janette, Lauren, Robert, and Meghan, for letting me follow my heart.

Stan Goldman, who coauthored my first book, *The Hand, Wrist, and Arm Sourcebook*, is not just a writer but a fascinating personality who made me aware of the need to inform the public about the hand. Writing requires a different kind of dedication than does surgery, and without his help I would never have been able to put pencil to paper. He has given me an intangible gift that I can never repay.

Thanks to Elaine Bammerlin, M.A., C.M.I., for her excellent line drawings.

Writing a book requires both thinking and doing. Joyce Strothman, my administrative assistant, came through for me when I felt as if I couldn't do another thing. In minutes, she was able to accomplish tasks that I couldn't bear to even start. I appreciate her work every day.

Monica Faulkner took our crude ideas and transformed them into something that was cohesive and readable. She did something I could not do, and I have the greatest respect for her expertise. I know about the hand, but without her help I would not have been able to pass this knowledge on to my readers. I've learned a lot from her, and I thank her for that as well.

Thanks to Rena Copperman, and others I haven't met. I hope that readers of this book will find answers and help for their hands.

PART ONE

Carpal Tunnel Syndrome: The Basics

Introduction

Carpal tunnel syndrome is one of the most interesting, controversial, and difficult hand problems in modern medicine. Put simply, carpal tunnel syndrome is a constellation of symptoms caused when a ˋnerve that travels through a small tunnel at the wrist becomes compressed or pinched.

It sounds so *simple*.

And it should be, except that attached to that hand and nerve is a person—a complicated, living, breathing, working human being who has problems with sleeping, bills, kids, the spouse, the boss . . . and when that person is having a problem with pain and numbness of the hand, carpal tunnel syndrome can interfere with much that makes life enjoyable.

As we'll see, carpal tunnel syndrome, though rooted in anatomy and physiology, is also affected by social and historical conditions and circumstances that all act in concert to make the problem vary in its presentation and outcome. As a physical condition, carpal tunnel syndrome is often relatively simple to treat, which is a relief to the patient and rewarding for the doctor. But when the standard treatments don't work, it can be difficult and frustrating.

Let's start with some basic definitions.

1 What is carpal tunnel syndrome?

Carpal *tunnel syndrome* is a medical condition defined as a group of symptoms caused by the compression of the median *nerve* located inside the *carpal tunnel* of each wrist.

This nerve, which transmits sensations from the fingers and hand to the brain, is vital for hand function. When it becomes pinched or compressed, the messages to the brain slow down and the brain interprets this as numbness. As we'll see, this problem is more common at night, when the numbness and discomfort can awaken people from sleep, sometimes repeatedly. Current medical treatments are designed to provide relief from the numbness and to improve the hand's functioning by reducing or eliminating the pinching of the nerve.

In the past twenty or so years, carpal tunnel syndrome has become a social and even political issue as well as a medical one, because it is one of a controversial group of medical difficulties that some believe are caused by conditions in today's workplaces.

2 Why do people get carpal tunnel syndrome?

No one really knows why some people get carpal tunnel syndrome and others do not. As we'll see, compression of the median nerve in the carpal tunnel has many causes, and most physicians and researchers believe that carpal tunnel syndrome is caused by many factors that act together to produce the symptoms. Most of the time, doctors can't attribute a patient's carpal tunnel syndrome to any one factor or, in fact, to anything obvious. In the medical profession, we say this is *idiopathic*, meaning that we just don't know the cause.

Some features that may act together to cause carpal tunnel syndrome include alterations in the body's fluid balance and our body position when we sleep. Sleeping positions often cause compression of the median nerve, and we're seldom aware of how we twist and bend our wrists during sleep.

We also know that carpal tunnel syndrome is more common among certain individuals, including diabetics and pregnant women, but in most cases it's hard to identify a specific cause.

3 *Why is it called a* syndrome?

A *syndrome* is a medical term for a collection of symptoms. *Symptoms* are unusual physical disturbances that patients notice about themselves and that send them to a doctor.

For example, in carpal tunnel syndrome, the main symptom is numbness of the hand and fingers. Physical findings, also called *signs*, are what your doctor notices when examining you. When your doctor taps on your wrist over the median nerve and causes an electrical sensation to race into your fingers, this is a sign.

Carpal tunnel syndrome as a condition is defined by the presence of a collection of symptoms and signs. Unlike other types of medical conditions, such as a fracture in which the broken bone is visible on an x ray or a tumor that is revealed in a biopsy, in a syndrome no single test or observation can definitively prove that the condition is present. Carpal tunnel syndrome gets its name because it is a collection of symptoms that is caused by compression of the median nerve in the carpal tunnel.

4 *What are the main symptoms of carpal tunnel syndrome?*

Numbness of the fingers, pain, and clumsiness in the hand are the three major symptoms of carpal tunnel syndrome, and numbness is the most important of the three. If you don't have numbness, you probably don't have carpal tunnel syndrome.

Although the numbness is usually felt in the thumb, index finger, long finger, and the lower half of the ring finger, you may feel numbness in the entire hand. We aren't sure why this is so. Perhaps the median nerve is so important that when its territory is numb, the brain perceives the whole hand as numb. Or, it could be that when the numbness awakens you at night, you're so sleepy that it feels as if your whole hand is involved. In any case, this numbness is notorious for waking up people. You may find that you want to shake your hand, hang it over the side of the bed, or run it under warm water to relieve the numbness. Shaking your hand when numbness awakens you at night is a very specific sign for carpal tunnel syndrome.

Numbness can also come on during other activities that require you to hold your wrist in a prolonged or exaggerated position either toward the *flexion* (inner) side or the *extension* (outer) side of the arm. Holding a telephone and grasping the steering wheel while driving are common examples.

Pain is another common symptom. You may perceive it as a burning or stabbing sensation that comes on with the numbness. At night, either the pain or the numbness can awaken you. Some patients experience pain in the inner side of the wrist or in the fingers, and some even report pain that radiates up the arm to the neck and shoulder. Because many different wrist, hand, and arm problems can cause pain, it's important that your doctor evaluate the cause of pain and recommend treatment. But if pain is your only symptom, you probably don't have carpal tunnel syndrome.

If you have the third common symptom, hand clumsiness, you may notice weakness or that you tend to drop things. Or you may perceive that you're not as dexterous in performing subtle motor activities such as fastening buttons or handling coins.

Because the median nerve provides power to the small muscles of the ball of the thumb, this clumsiness may be due to the weakening of those muscles. It's also possible that the decrease in sensation caused by the compression of the median nerve reduces your perception of how you're holding objects. That lack of sensory feedback may in turn result in clumsiness.

In early carpal tunnel syndrome, the symptoms are intermittent, but if nerve compression is prolonged or severe, the numbness and pain can become more intense, more frequent, or even constant.

5 How serious are these symptoms?

In some conditions, symptoms are a warning sign of a potentially dangerous illness. For example, you're no doubt aware that angina—a dull, squeezing pain in the central chest—can be a symptom of a heart attack. The chest pain itself may not be pleasant, but its presence as an indicator of damage to the heart is serious. It's the heart damage that's life threatening, not the symptom of chest pain.

In carpal tunnel syndrome, the pain or numbness that awakens you at night is a symptom that suggests that the median nerve is being compressed. Your symptoms are serious to the degree that they cause discomfort, limit the use of your hands, or interfere with your sleep. And if treatment relieves those symptoms, then your carpal tunnel syndrome is being effectively addressed. In other words, when it comes to carpal tunnel syndrome, the goal of the treatment is to relieve the symptoms, because if the compression is cured, you won't have any more symptoms.

From another perspective, carpal tunnel syndrome can be considered a serious condition because it may require surgery, and any problem that requires surgery is serious by definition. Fortunately, however, carpal tunnel surgery is much less extensive and invasive than many other types of surgery.

6 What activities cause the symptoms of carpal tunnel syndrome?

As mentioned in Question 4, any activity that requires your wrist to remain in an exaggerated flexed or extended position for a long period of time can bring on the symptoms of carpal tunnel syndrome.

As we'll see in Part Four, which discusses employment and work-related activities, it's difficult to know whether these activities cause carpal tunnel syndrome. Occupations that require repetitive gripping of the fingers (for example, the use of pistol-grip power guns) are controversial. This is discussed in more detail in Questions 31 and 32.

Even more controversial is the possible relationship between carpal tunnel syndrome and using a computer keyboard and computer mouse. Unfortunately, these are areas of great uncertainty, and only time and research will be able to clarify the relationships between these specific job activities and carpal tunnel syndrome.

Also, Part Nine, Question 99, touches on the possible relationships among various sports and carpal tunnel syndrome.

7 Is carpal tunnel syndrome the only cause of hand numbness?

Although numbness is the main symptom of carpal tunnel syndrome and carpal tunnel syndrome is probably the most frequent cause of numbness, medical conditions of the peripheral and central nervous system can also cause this problem. For example, one common symptom of diabetes is numbness in the hands and feet.

In addition, compression of major nerves can cause numbness. The nerves that transmit sensations to the fingers can become compressed at many locations from the spine, along the shoulders, and down the arms to the wrists. Compression at any one or more of these sites, other than the carpal tunnel, can also cause finger numbness. The most common of these conditions will be discussed in Part Two.

If you're experiencing numbness, your best course of action is to have your doctor carry out a thorough medical examination and evaluation so that you can rule out any more serious conditions and also determine whether your numbness is due to carpal tunnel syndrome or to compression at any other site.

8 What other conditions can be confused with carpal tunnel syndrome?

A number of hand, arm, and even shoulder conditions not related to the median nerve can cause symptoms that resemble those of carpal tunnel syndrome.

As mentioned, the median nerve can be compressed at other locations in the upper limb, which can cause symptoms that mimic carpal tunnel syndrome. Also, other nerves such as the ulnar nerve in the elbow can be compressed, which may cause symptoms that resemble carpal tunnel syndrome. The most common of these conditions are examined in more detail in Part Two.

Understanding the Hand:
Anatomy and Physiology

Introduction

Anatomy is the body of knowledge of the bones, nerves, ligaments, and other structures that make up the human body. *Physiology* studies how the parts of the body act and what chemical, biological, and other processes keep them going. For hand surgeons, anatomy focuses on the structure of the hand because it provides a road map for any kind of treatment and surgery, while physiology offers knowledge of how the hand should function and what may be keeping it from doing so.

The importance of anatomy and physiology goes far beyond knowing your way around the ligaments, nerves, and bones, however. They are both codes that tell you and your doctor how the hand works, how things can go wrong, and how the hand can be repaired. Deciphering the hand and its mysteries requires logic, common sense, and awareness of other sciences, including mechanics, physics, and biology.

When it comes to the hand, the links between anatomy and function are obvious: the fingers flex to hold an object; the index fingertip and the pad of the thumb come together to feel a small object. At a deeper level, we can see more—a lot more. For example, the joint at the base of the thumb is a saddle shape that allows it an incredible range of motion in all directions. Another example is the *scaphoid bone*, which straddles the first and second rows of the wrist bones. It creates stability and yet allows the wrist to move. The more closely we look, the more we see the incredible linkages between the hand's anatomy, or form, and its functioning. One does not determine the other; they're completely meshed and interdependent.

If you want to see how the hand works, study its anatomy; and the more carefully you study its anatomy, the more profoundly you'll understand its functioning. Also, the more you study the hand's function, the better you'll understand how its anatomy can be repaired and reconstructed after injury or disease. We surgeons have a history of trying to solve difficult problems by careful study of anatomy because we believe that the more thoroughly we understand it, the more likely we are to find solutions.

And yet, beyond the links between form and function, beautiful though these are, lies something more, something deeper. I believe that there's a "master plan" for the hand. Whether this master plan is due to divine intervention or to the grueling struggle of evolution over millions of years, the anatomy of the hand contains within it a brilliant plan for function and survival.

Consider first that there are two large arteries, not just one, that provide life-giving blood flow to the hand, and two arteries that go to each finger. This built-in redundancy minimizes the chance of your losing a hand or a finger if one of the arteries becomes injured or blocked due to disease.

Another example: Where do the nerves of your hand lie? Under the palm, its most protected area. In addition to the two arteries, each finger has two nerves, and the location and anatomy of these nerves indicate a careful plan for protection and preservation from possible injury. The nerves that transmit sensation from the adjacent sides of the fingers branch from common nerves called the *common palmar digital nerve* so that no single finger is supplied by only one nerve. If you cut one of those nerves in the palm area, your whole finger won't become numb. Rather, you'll lose sensation in only half of each of the two affected fingers.

The answers to many questions about carpal tunnel syndrome are to be found in the anatomy of the hand, wrist, and forearm. To understand the hand's anatomy and functioning is to understand the hand.

9 *What is the carpal tunnel, and how did it get that name?*

The carpal tunnel is an actual physical tunnel made up of bones and a fibrous band of tissue located at the wrist. On the inner or flexion side of your wrist (the hairless side), the wrist bones create the concave side

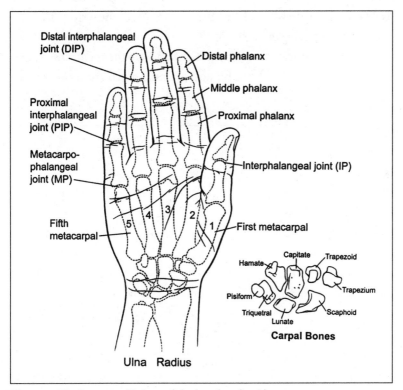

Figure 1. The bones and joints of the hand and wrist

of an arch. Figure 1 shows the bones and joints of the hand and wrist in relation to the lower ends of the two bones in the forearm, the *radius* and the *ulna*. Anatomic structures such as tendons, fingers, and nerves that lie on the same side of the hand as the radius are called *radial* in their position, and structures on the same side as the ulna are called *ulnar*.

The carpal tunnel is a bony concavity, usually about 3 cm by 2 cm, made up of eight *carpal bones* that form the "floor" of the tunnel, which actually lies on the outer (hairy) side of the wrist, and the "walls" on either side of the wrist. The "roof" of the carpal tunnel is made up of a strong, wide ligament called the *transverse carpal ligament* (sometimes called the *flexor retinaculum*), which runs across the wrist just beneath the skin on the palm side of your hand (see Figure 2). If you hold a pen as if you're going to write a letter, the flexion side of the wrist will be the side facing or resting on the table.

Other anatomical structures in the hand are the *metacarpals*, five bones that run across the palm and are numbered from one to five

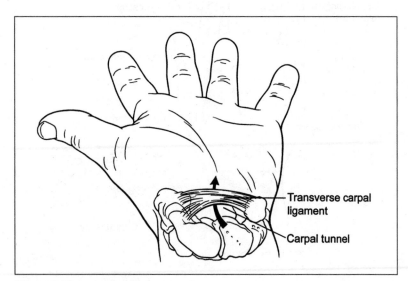

Figure 2. The carpal tunnel

starting with the thumb. The finger bones (*phalanges* is the plural term and *phalanx* is the singular) are linked to the metacarpals. The thumb has only two phalanges, and each of the four fingers has three. Figure 1 also shows the web of soft tissue between each finger that starts about halfway down the length of the first phalanx.

Figure 2 shows how the carpal tunnel bones and transverse carpal ligament form the carpal tunnel. Various physical structures pass through the carpal tunnel and into the hand, as indicated by the arrow. These structures include the nine *flexor tendons,* which help the digits to move, and the *median nerve.* Figure 2 makes it clear that because the carpal tunnel bones are rigid, there's no room for expansion, so any increase in the size of the structures inside it can cause compression of the softest structure, which is the median nerve.

The term *carpal tunnel* is derived from *carpus,* the Greek word for "wrist." Most medical conditions relating to the wrist will include the term *carpal*; a broken wrist bone is a *carpal fracture* and a wrist splint is called a *carpal splint.*

10 *What is the median nerve, and what does it do?*

The median nerve is usually about a quarter of an inch wide, or about the width of a lead pencil. Like other nerves, it acts as a two-way highway for transmitting electrical information to and from the brain. Most nerves serve two functions: sensory functions that transmit sensations from the skin to the brain and motor functions that innervate muscles or send messages to muscles to move.

The median nerve picks up sensory information from the thumbs, the index and long fingers, and the radial half of the ring fingers and transmits that information through small biological electrical "cables," called *axons,* up the arm to the spinal cord and then to the brain. In the forearm, the median nerve also innervates some of the muscles that flex the fingers and the wrist (see Question 11). In other words, when the brain wills the hand to move, the electrical signals start in the brain and are transmitted through the nerve to the muscles, which then contract and move the joints.

There are two other major nerves in the arm: the ulnar nerve and the radial nerve. All three major nerves originate from the spinal cord in the region of the neck just above the collarbone, where they are part of a complicated intermingling of nerves called the *brachial plexus.* From this intermingling, the nerves sort themselves into the three large nerves.

Figure 3 shows the radial, ulnar, and median nerves, along with their origin at the neck and their intermingling in the brachial plexus. The median nerve travels along the inside of the upper arm, crosses in front of the elbow, moves down the forearm deep beneath the superfi-

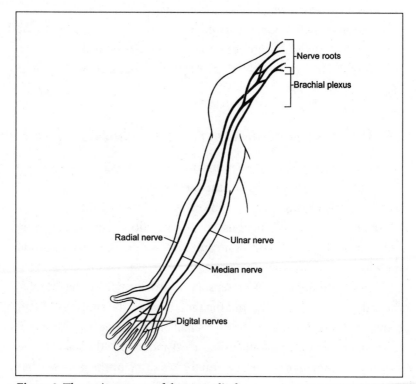

Figure 3. The major nerves of the upper limb

cial flexor muscles, and emerges just above the wrist bones, where it enters the carpal tunnel along with the tendons that flex the fingers and the thumb. (Note that because it's so close to the surface in this region, it is susceptible to injury.)

After it emerges from the carpal tunnel into the palm, the median nerve branches into the five smaller common palmar digital nerves. One large branch, about the diameter of the lead in a standard pencil, curves around the edge of the muscles of the ball of the thumb and provides power for those muscles.

Two of the five branches go to the thumb, while three others make their way to the index finger, the long (middle) finger, and half of the ring finger to provide sensation to these digits. These digital nerve branches lie along the sides of the fingers and thumb and have several smaller branches to various areas on the digits. Although other, smaller nerves branch from the median nerve after it emerges from the carpal tunnel, the ones mentioned here are the largest and most important.

The ulnar and radial nerves power other parts of the hand and arm. The ulnar nerve sits behind the elbow in a groove between the point of the elbow and the *medial epicondyle,* the bump on the inside of your elbow. Because of its location, this nerve is susceptible to minor trauma and is often bumped, which causes an electrical signal to race down to the hand. The so-called funny bone isn't a bone at all; it is actually the ulnar nerve.

The ulnar nerve moves down the arm toward the hand through the forearm and the heel side of the hand. It gives feeling to the little finger and the upper (ulnar) half of the ring finger. In addition, most of the small muscles of the hand receive their power from the ulnar nerve. For example, it controls the muscles that perform many activities requiring dexterity. When you roll a ball in the palm of your hand, the ulnar nerve is at work. The ulnar nerve doesn't go through the carpal tunnel and isn't affected by carpal tunnel syndrome, but sometimes ulnar nerve problems can cause symptoms that patients confuse with

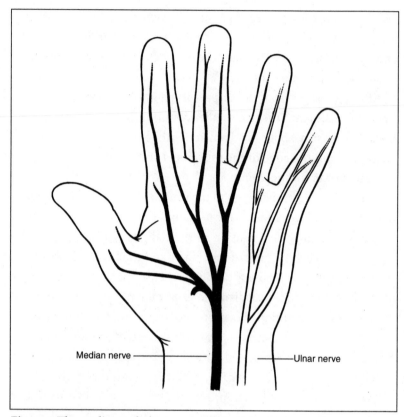

Median nerve

Ulnar nerve

Figure 4. The median and ulnar nerves

carpal tunnel syndrome. Figure 4 illustrates the position of the median and ulnar nerves in the hand.

The common digital nerves in the palm give feeling to the adjacent sides of two fingers. For this reason, mentioned earlier, if one nerve in the palm is cut, an entire finger will not lose sensation.

The radial nerve (shown only in Figure 3) lies on the outside of the arm and innervates the muscles that extend the elbow, such as the triceps, as well as those that extend the wrist, the thumb, and the large knuckles of the fingers. It carries sensation from the back of the hand to the brain.

11 *What do nerves do?*

Nerves are biological "electrical cables" made up of living cells, the basic building blocks that make up all of life. The nerve cell body of a peripheral nerve is located within or adjacent to the spinal cord and has short extensions that connect to the spinal cord. The axons, long extensions of the cell body that reach from the cell body to skin and muscle all over the body, are two-way highways that provide control of the muscles and transmit sensory information from the skin to the brain. The cell body is like a factory that produces biochemical transmitters to deliver messages to the ends of the nerves.

Each peripheral nerve is made up of a large number of sensory and motor axons that transmit information and chemical transmitters. Peripheral nerves are composed of many types of tissue, including blood vessels, collagen, and others, but two specific types of tissue that are seen in the peripheral nerve are the axon and *Schwann cells.* Schwann cells are supportive cells for the axon and produce myelin insulation for the nerve. It's probably easiest to think of the nerve as an electrical cable with axons being the copper wire and Schwann cells providing the insulation.

At the end of the axon of the motor nerve component, the nerve makes contact with muscle through microscopic connections called *synapses.* When a message travels down the nerve to make the muscle move, a chemical signal jumps the microscopic distance at the synapse and stimulates the muscle to contract.

Signals for sensory information are picked up by special receptors in the skin and transmitted through specific sensory nerves to the spinal cord and up to the brain.

The sensory receptors in our skin are exquisitely sensitive. For example, our fingertips are so sensitive that we can distinguish tiny 2- to 4-micron–sized dots on a flat glass plate just by stroking the dot with the pads of our fingers. In addition, researchers at Massachusetts Institute of Technology have shown that the nerves within our finger-pads are sensitive to changes in the curvature of cylindrical objects of just a few millimeters.

12 What is the transverse carpal ligament, and why is it so important?

As described earlier in Question 9, the transverse carpal ligament, or flexor retinaculum, forms the roof of the carpal tunnel. It acts as a pulley for the tendons that flex the fingers.

When you hold your wrist in a flexed position, the tendons try to move away from the bones of the wrist, but the ligament holds them against the bones and prevents them from "bowing out" away from the bones. If the transverse carpal ligament were not present, the tendons would push up directly against the underside of the skin, and they would also lose a lot of their mechanical strength. The job of the transverse carpal ligament is to hold the tendons close to the wrist joint. This gives them the most efficient mechanical opportunity to move the fingers.

In carpal tunnel surgery, often referred to as carpal tunnel release, the surgeon severs the transverse carpal ligament, which enlarges the carpal tunnel and creates more room for the median nerve and the tendons. After carpal tunnel surgery, the cut edges of the ligament heal back together but leave about 25 percent more space in the tunnel. This, in turn, relieves pressure on the median nerve and results in relief from symptoms.

Figure 5 shows the median nerve as it travels through the carpal tunnel. Two of the nine tubelike flexor tendons that also travel through the carpal tunnel are shown here to indicate their size relative to the median nerve. The figure shows the transverse carpal ligament with its origin and insertion from the carpal bones as it forms the roof of the carpal tunnel. The major branches of the median nerve start just past the tunnel in the palm of the hand. As mentioned earlier, the median nerve branches to govern both sides of the thumb, the index finger, and the middle finger, as well as the side of the ring finger closest to the middle finger. Each finger has two digital nerves, one on either side.

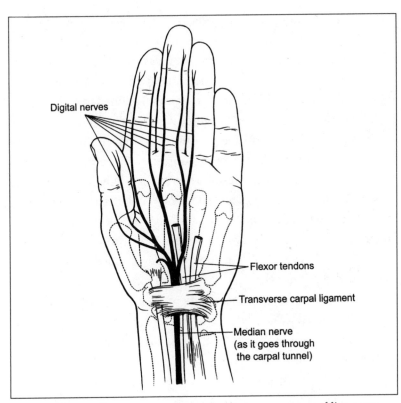

Figure 5. The median nerve passing under the transverse carpal ligament

13 What is nerve compression, and why is it believed to cause carpal tunnel syndrome?

Nerve compression describes what people commonly call a "pinched nerve." As mentioned earlier, when a nerve is compressed or pinched, it is less able to transmit messages to and from the brain. Our brains interpret this as numbness, and we perceive weakness or clumsiness.

Prolonged nerve compression can cause anatomic changes or damage to the structure of the nerve and result in more severe symptoms. Also, numbness can become constant, and the muscles affected by the nerve can atrophy or shrink. This problem is called *wasting*.

Research findings in several studies support the idea that compression of the median nerve causes carpal tunnel syndrome. In a number of studies, researchers placed pressure-measuring devices inside the carpal tunnel of healthy volunteers and patients with carpal tunnel syndrome. Pressure within the carpal tunnel seemed to be higher in patients with symptoms than in people with no symptoms.

Other studies have compared pressure measurements when patients with carpal tunnel syndrome and volunteers in a control group place their wrists in positions that are known to increase symptoms. Here, too, pressures in the carpal tunnel increased. We'll look at one such position, Phalen's test, in Part Five, when we discuss what your doctor will do when you have your carpal tunnel syndrome symptoms assessed (see Question 45 and Figure 7). In Phalen's test, the wrist is flexed with the fingers pointing toward the inner (hairless) side of the forearm. This position is known to bring on carpal tunnel symptoms in susceptible patients.

Finally, when doctors study the nerve during carpal tunnel surgery, they can see that it looks pinched, especially in patients with severe carpal tunnel syndrome.

Other evidence also points to pressure or compression as the cause of carpal tunnel syndrome. For example, lesions or tumors that grow and take up space in the carpal tunnel will cause the typical symptoms of carpal tunnel syndrome. Although these conditions are very rare, they indicate that when the carpal tunnel gets tight, symptoms of carpal tunnel syndrome will arise. Conversely, after the tumor or other mass in the carpal tunnel is removed and the pressure on the nerve is relieved, the symptoms of carpal tunnel syndrome decrease and even disappear.

14 How does compression or pressure interfere with the functioning of the median nerve?

Like all other tissues in our bodies, nerves need nutrition to survive and to function properly. They receive nutrition through the circulatory system. Our arteries bring blood to our tissues, and our veins return the "used" blood to our hearts.

When a nerve is compressed, even slightly, the compression blocks the drainage of blood into the veins. Meanwhile, the arterial blood continues to flow into the nerve at a higher pressure. This pressure causes the nerve to swell and impairs its ability to conduct electrical signals to and from the brain. If the pressure is prolonged or becomes more severe, the very physical architecture of the nerve can be damaged. For example, the myelin, or protective sheath that insulates the nerve, can become deformed. With severe or prolonged compression, the axons, or electrical "cables" within the nerve that transmit electrical signals, can atrophy to the point where they simply disappear, or, in medical terms, *drop out.*

If the pressure has impaired the ability of the veins to drain blood from the nerve, relieving that pressure through surgery can reverse the impairment very quickly. Some patients experience immediate relief from hand numbness right after surgery. However, if the myelin has been damaged or deformed, or if axons have dropped out, even relieving the pressure through surgery may not result in complete recovery of the nerve.

There are many possible sources of increased pressure that can cause carpal tunnel syndrome. The most common cause is posture of the hand. Certain positions, such as flexion and extension of the wrist, are known to increase the pressure in the carpal tunnel. Fluid imbalances in the body, which may be present in patients with kidney problems or some types of heart disease, can result in increased fluid in the carpal tunnel and hence increased pressure. Any type of swelling, such as that caused by inflammation, can also increase carpal tunnel pressure. Rheumatoid arthritis is a common cause of inflammation in the carpal tunnel, while masses and tumors, though rare, can cause increased pressure.

15 Why do my hands go to sleep at night?

There are two explanations for this common symptom of carpal tunnel syndrome. Remember, numbness is caused by compression of the median nerve in the tunnel. Because there's no extra room in the tunnel, anything that makes the space tighter can cause carpal tunnel syndrome.

During the day, the fluid that circulates within our bodies is affected by gravity. (Like other parts of the body, everything "gravitates" downward, as we all realize only too well when age starts creeping up on us.) It's a well-known fact that our body fluid moves from the upper body to the legs when we're on our feet all day. Some patients with heart failure or kidney problems, which can cause excess fluid retention, find that their ankles swell by the end of the day, partly for this reason. Chest x-rays taken when patients are standing show more fluid in the lower parts of the lungs than in the upper lung areas. In contrast, conditions of weightlessness, such as those experienced by astronauts on the space shuttle and during other journeys into space, cause more fluid to stay in astronauts' upper bodies, with a variety of consequences that include back pain, headaches, and facial swelling.

When we lie down, we still have extra fluid in our legs, but as soon as we put up our legs, gravity stops pulling fluid into them. The body fluids gets redistributed more evenly and flow into the upper body and hands. If the carpal tunnels are already tight, the additional fluid can compress the nerve enough that the brain perceives numbness, and that's what wakes you up. So we believe that there is a connection between carpal tunnel syndrome and gravity's effect on body fluid.

The second reason for nighttime numbness is the posture of our hands when we sleep. We know from pressure measurements taken inside the carpal tunnel that pressure in the tunnel is greater when the wrist is flexed or extended than when it's held straight. Many people sleep with their wrists either partially flexed or partially extended, and extremes in either of these positions may put pressure on the carpal tunnel and cause the numbness that wakes you up at night. As will be explained in Part Five, that's why one of the first treatments recommended for carpal tunnel syndrome is to wear a splint at night—it keeps your wrists straight while you're sleeping.

16 What is inflammation, and can it cause carpal tunnel syndrome?

Inflammation is a basic mechanism that the body uses to deal with tissue injury. When you injure yourself in any way, an automatic process begins in your body for handling and healing the injury. Chemical messages from the area of the injury cause the blood vessels to dilate, which allows more blood to flow to the area of the injury. The increased blood flow creates redness in the area. The increased circulation and chemical mediators in the area also cause warmth. Small blood vessels in the area of the injury begin to leak slightly, which allows tissue fluid, white blood cells, and protein to leak into the tissue. This leakage causes swelling. Some of the chemical mediators in the tissue cause pain, which will cause you to reduce your use of the injured part or area.

So it should be clear that inflammation can cause carpal tunnel syndrome. Because swelling is one facet of inflammation, inflammation in the carpal tunnel can decrease the space in the tunnel and compress the median nerve.

17 Why would tissue injury occur in the carpal tunnel?

I use the term *tissue injury* in a very general sense when speaking about carpal tunnel syndrome because most patients with the condition don't have inflammation in the carpal tunnel. Many factors can create pressure on the nerve.

Among the less common causes of carpal tunnel syndrome are certain types of arthritis, rare types of infection, and other disease processes that can cause inflammation in the carpal tunnel, and because of the swelling caused by the inflammation, cause symptoms of carpal tunnel syndrome. Osteoarthritis can cause "bone spurs" to develop in the carpal tunnel, and the movement of tendons over these spurs can wear down the tendons until they rupture. Then the ruptured, inflamed ends of the tendon lying in the carpal tunnel can cause swelling, resulting in carpal tunnel syndrome.

Trauma to the area of the carpal tunnel can cause injury to the median nerve and result in acute carpal tunnel syndrome. When I was a young surgeon, I struck my wrist on the tip of a water ski during a fall. For thirty minutes afterward, the fingers served by the median nerve were completely numb because I had bruised it so severely. Fortunately, the nerve recovered within a short time, but if the contusion had caused serious swelling, it might also have resulted in my developing acute carpal tunnel syndrome.

18 What is cubital tunnel syndrome, and is it related to carpal tunnel syndrome?

The cubital tunnel is the tunnel behind the inside of the elbow. The ulnar nerve runs down from the shoulder, through the cubital tunnel, and down the arm to the ulnar side of the hand. As mentioned earlier, it serves the ulnar side of the ring finger and both sides of the little finger.

Like the median nerve, the ulnar nerve can become compressed. The symptoms of cubital tunnel syndrome are numbness in the small and ring fingers and clumsiness of the hand. The symptoms of cubital tunnel syndrome typically occur when your elbow is bent, and, like carpal tunnel syndrome, can wake you up at night. Your doctor can recommend a range of treatments if your diagnosis is cubital tunnel syndrome.

19 What is thoracic outlet syndrome?

Thoracic outlet syndrome is a complex form of nerve compression in the region of the neck where the collarbone crosses over the first rib; it is sometimes difficult to diagnose. I've already discussed how the large nerves that carry information to and from the arms and the spinal cord and then the brain are involved in the complicated arrangement called the brachial plexus (see Question 10).

Because this region is crowded, some doctors believe that the nerves of the brachial plexus can become compressed there. Also, we know that anatomic variations in the muscles, such as the *scalenes,* in this area, or injuries such as a broken collarbone that fails to heal properly, can compress the nerves. Aneurysms of the major blood vessels of the neck can also compress these nerves and have been known to cause thoracic outlet syndrome. Depending on which nerves are compressed, patients can experience numbness either on the side of the hand where symptoms of carpal tunnel syndrome are felt or on the ulnar side of the hand.

Thoracic outlet syndrome is sometimes considered a controversial diagnosis because it's hard to prove beyond a doubt that the nerves in that area are compressed. *Electrodiagnostic testing,* discussed in Part Five, isn't reliable in the brachial plexus because of the large number of nerves in the area that can transmit the signal and confuse the interpretation of the results. In addition, the findings from physical examination of this area are more difficult to interpret.

Surgical treatment for this condition has not been as successful as decompression for pinched nerves in other locations, leading some doctors to wonder whether decompression surgery should be considered in any except the clearest cases.

Evaluating and treating patients with complex nerve compression problems in the hands and arms may require a team approach that includes a surgeon, a neurologist, a physical therapist, and possibly other specialists as well. In the absence of a clear anatomic injury, however, all available forms of nonsurgical treatment should be tried before surgery is considered.

20 Can the median nerve be compressed in other areas besides the carpal tunnel?

The most common area outside the carpal tunnel where the median nerve can be compressed is in the midforearm, where it runs underneath the *pronator teres* muscle. For this reason, compression in this area is called *pronator syndrome,* a constellation of symptoms that resemble those produced by carpal tunnel syndrome. As shown in Figure 3, the path of the median nerve as it runs from the brachial plexus down the arm to the carpal tunnel takes it under the muscles that twist and flex the wrist and flex the fingers.

Repeated twisting and gripping motions can cause those forearm muscles to grow larger, sometimes large enough to compress the median nerve. In addition, in some patients the leading edge of the pronator muscle forms a fibrous sharp edge that may impinge on and compress the median nerve. Again, this condition can cause symptoms similar to carpal tunnel syndrome. In fact, the symptoms can be so similar that doctors find it hard to differentiate whether they're caused by carpal tunnel syndrome or pronator syndrome.

Figure 6 shows the common areas where nerve compression occurs in the upper limb.

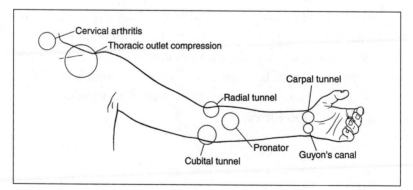

Figure 6. Common areas of nerve compression

To make the situation even more complicated, sometimes the median nerve or other nerves may be compressed at more than one location simultaneously. When a nerve is compressed at two sites in the arm, we say that a patient is suffering from *double crush syndrome.* And if the nerve is pinched at more than two locations, we use the term *multiple crush.*

There's some debate within the medical community about whether these complex forms of nerve compression actually exist, but I and my colleagues have seen many patients with symptoms and physical findings that are compatible with compression at more than one location. As you can imagine, the uncertainties and variations in symptoms, physical examination, treatment, and treatment results make this a difficult area to sort out. When we see patients who appear to have nerve compression at more than one location, we must look at all the major nerves from the neck down to the hand to try to understand what condition may be causing the symptoms.

When patients are suffering from apparent nerve compression in multiple locations, doctors often treat the carpal tunnel first because it's the most accessible, and because carpal tunnel surgery is less involved than surgery at other sites of nerve compression.

21 I've heard that arthritis of the neck can cause numbness of the hand. Is this true?

The major nerves that carry sensation from the hand pass through the sides of the spinal vertebrae through openings called *foramina* (the singular term is *foramen*) and connect to nerves in the spinal cord. The vertebrae are separated from each other by disks of fibrous material called *intervertebral disks* that are about the size and shape of a marshmallow cut in half.

It's possible that arthritis in the neck, which can come on with age or injury, can cause bony prominences, commonly called *bone spurs,* to form on the vertebrae. This can cause the foramina to narrow, which reduces the space through which nerves pass. If the nerves that pass down to the hands become compressed, this can lead to numbness, tingling, pain, and weakness—the same symptoms produced by other forms of nerve compression, including carpal tunnel syndrome.

The situation is even more complicated because we have medical evidence that compression of the nerves in the neck region, called the *cervical spine* in medical terminology, makes the nerves more susceptible to compression farther down the arm and in the carpal tunnel. Why is this the case? Because, as mentioned earlier, the axon of a single nerve cell extends all the way from the spinal cord to the fingertip.

We believe that when nerve compression slows the flow of electrical information and chemical transmitters among the hands and the brain, the median nerve becomes more sensitive to compression in another location—just as when you step on a garden hose, you reduce the flow of water all the way down to the nozzle.

Most adults who are middle aged and older will have some degree of arthritis of the neck, so it's important to consider this possibility in patients with nerve compression, especially those with nerve compression in multiple locations. People often report pain and grinding sensations in the neck region when they move their necks in certain directions. They also notice that symptoms worsen with certain activities and with straining, such as when lifting a weight. It is important to identify nerve compression at the cervical spine because it can cause symptoms similar to carpal tunnel syndrome.

22 *How do doctors diagnose nerve compression due to arthritis in the neck or the cervical spine?*

When a patient reports symptoms in the neck or symptoms that might indicate a pinched nerve, the standard approach is always to first obtain a medical history and then carry out a physical examination that will help the doctor localize the problem.

For example, if the patient reports symptoms in both hands, the doctor may suspect that the problem is originating, at least to some degree, in the neck rather than in the hands. The doctor may also suspect neck problems if the patient has had an injury in a motor vehicle collision and reports pain in the neck, stiffness, or grinding or clicking with movement.

During the physical examination, the doctor checks the motion of the patient's neck and notes any worsening of the symptoms. x-rays may also be taken to obtain a picture of the general condition of the neck. x-rays may also reveal areas of suspected nerve compression. Because the nerves travel through foramina, if the x-rays reveal any narrowing of these vital spaces, it suggests that the nerves that traverse these openings could be pinched.

In recent years, *magnetic resonance imaging,* commonly referred to as *MRI,* has become the main procedure for imaging the neck. MRIs use a strong magnetic field rather than x-rays to produce a picture of the internal structure of the body and can provide clear pictures of many of the neck's structures, including the spine and spinal cord.

Because compressions of the spinal cord and the major nerves in the region of the spine are potentially dangerous, you should have any symptoms of nerve compression evaluated by a physician.

23 Are conditions that cause pain but not numbness related to carpal tunnel syndrome?

As mentioned earlier, without numbness, you don't have carpal tunnel syndrome.

That said, a number of other medical conditions can certainly create discomfort in the carpal tunnel region. *De Quervain's tenosynovitis,* an inflammation of the *abductor pollicus longus* and *extensor pollicus brevis* tendons that straighten the thumb, causes pain on the thumb side of the wrist. This condition can be confused with carpal tunnel syndrome because these tendons are located near but outside the carpal tunnel.

Arthritis of the wrist or the base of the thumb (*basal joint arthritis*) can also cause pain and interfere with your ability to use your hand. These conditions cause pain but do not in themselves cause numbness.

It's sometimes hard to differentiate among the various conditions that can cause hand symptoms. A hand surgeon is the medical specialist best trained to make an accurate diagnosis and to suggest the most effective treatment.

PART THREE

History and Epidemiology: Carpal Tunnel Syndrome over Time and in Populations

Introduction

Epidemiology is the study of how illnesses, diseases, and medical conditions appear in populations over time and in different societies and social subgroups. By studying the epidemiology of a disease, we can learn about causes; variations; treatment successes, failures, and costs; and prevention.

Our Western medical model accepts a "disease-oriented" model of health in which "to be healthy" means "to be free of disease." Over the years, the medical profession has come up with what I call "packages" of disease, constellations of symptoms that are thought to have similar causes and can be cured by using treatments that have been shown to work. So your doctor will tell you that you have such-and-such a disease or illness or condition and that such-and-such a treatment will cure it and get it out of your body. If your package of disease is common and looks the same as packages present in many other people, doctors have no trouble recognizing it and using their training and experience to give you treatment that will rid you of the disease and make you healthy again. Luckily, most health problems appear in a more or less typical fashion and are easy to recognize.

Epidemiology has also helped us to realize that certain health problems are relatively predictable, given the human life cycle. This is similar to the situation with cars. Mechanics may know that the transmission of a certain make of car typically goes out at around 80,000 miles. Similarly, doctors know that by the age of fifty or so most people have developed at least some arthritis in the base of the thumb.

Now let's introduce some variability. Not all people are the same. Not all hands are the same, and not all medical problems come in the same easily identifiable package. Variety may be the spice of life, but it can also be the undoing of Western medicine. Suppose that your disease package is a little different from everyone else's. Your doctor may recognize it as one of the natural variations of the disease and still give you the correct treatment. But if your package is so different that your doctor has trouble recognizing it, you may not get the appropriate treatment, and you won't be returned to good health. Finally, if your package is completely unrecognizable, you may go into the land of "I don't know," or maybe the doctor will invent a package for your problem that will someday become another recognized condition. In fact, some doctors believe that this is how the concept of *repetitive strain injuries* has come to be invented.

Epidemiology is important because it gives us the "big picture" that we would never be able to grasp by examining just one specific patient with one specific set of symptoms. It gives us statistical regularities and general tendencies that apply across relatively large numbers of people.

So when it comes to carpal tunnel syndrome, we can't resolve the questions about links with assembly-line work, computer keyboards, gender, other diseases, or other factors based on one single patient. We must look at larger populations of patients and people.

Today we have good tests for carpal tunnel syndrome, we have excellent treatments for carpal tunnel syndrome, we have a lot of experience, and we know how to take care of patients with carpal tunnel syndrome. Still, if you have carpal tunnel syndrome and you wonder whether it is because you use a computer keyboard or work on an assembly line or engage in some other activity, no one can tell you with 100 percent certainty. All we can do is look at the epidemiological evidence.

This section also looks at the history of carpal tunnel syndrome. Although this condition has become part of our everyday terminology only in the past twenty or so years, it has existed as a medically recognized condition since the mid-nineteenth century. Medical history is informative and important because it shows us the building blocks of knowledge on which current treatments are based. The lens of history is a powerful way to clarify what is happening in the present.

24 How many people have carpal tunnel syndrome?

This is a difficult question to answer precisely, partly because the incidence or frequency of the condition depends on how you define carpal tunnel syndrome. Many people have symptoms in their hands that are not severe enough to cause them to go to a doctor. Some of these people may have mild carpal tunnel syndrome, but they are not counted statistically if they do not seek treatment.

When measured by the number of patients who are having enough problems with their hands to see a doctor, the prevalence of diagnosed carpal tunnel syndrome is estimated at about one in a thousand.

I estimate, however, that if all adults with any symptoms—mild, moderate, or severe—were taken into account, the prevalence might be as much as 4 percent of the general population. I should note that carpal tunnel syndrome is very rare in children but can occur as the result of a congenital variation that causes pinching of the median nerve.

Carpal tunnel syndrome is more common in certain defined populations, such as pregnant women (see Questions 25 and 68) (perhaps because of fluid changes in the body during pregnancy) and among people engaged in certain occupational categories, but once again the exact prevalence is not known because of variations in how the condition is diagnosed and the ways that various populations have been evaluated.

25 What population groups are most susceptible to carpal tunnel syndrome?

This is a fascinating question that touches on the changes in the epidemiology of the disease. Demographic data regarding age at onset of carpal tunnel syndrome has changed somewhat over the past few decades, and its relationship with work activity has changed as well.

In the 1950s and 1960s, when the condition first became commonly recognized, it was a disease of those in their forties and fifties and seemed to afflict mostly homemakers and patients with certain medical conditions, such as rheumatoid arthritis.

By the 1970s and 1980s, the problem seemed to be occurring more commonly among machine and assembly-line workers, thus encompassing more younger patients and an increasing number of men.

And in the 1990s, the demographic pattern shifted again, as computer keyboard work came under suspicion as a probable cause of carpal tunnel syndrome.

Today, we still have no clear, widely accepted explanation for these shifts in the age at onset or the causes of carpal tunnel syndrome. We do know that it affects adults of all ages, for we're seeing patients ranging in age from the early twenties to the eighties.

As mentioned earlier, carpal tunnel syndrome is a common condition in pregnancy, perhaps due to increased fluid volume or to changes in sleep postures that put pressure on the wrist and median nerve. It's also common in patients with specific medical problems such as rheumatoid arthritis, and among those who have suffered injuries such as a fracture of the *distal radius,* commonly called a broken wrist.

Historically, carpal tunnel syndrome is twice as common among women as men, and this is still true today. We don't have a clear explanation for this. It may be related to the fact that most women's wrists, and thus their carpal tunnels, are smaller than most men's, or to other physiological or anatomical factors that we haven't yet discovered. Also, statistics show that women tend to consult doctors more often than men do, and of course only women become pregnant.

But most patients with carpal tunnel syndrome are just like you and me, regular folks who for no obvious reason develop numbness of their hands, mostly at night.

26 Is carpal tunnel syndrome inherited?

If we're very lucky, we may have an answer to this question in another two or three decades. Because carpal tunnel syndrome did not become widely recognized until the 1950s and 1960s, we haven't had enough experience with it or collected enough data to know whether it is an inherited condition. We'll need another generation of research and record keeping to evaluate this issue.

27 Is there any way to predict who will get carpal tunnel syndrome?

Some injuries, such as distal radius or other wrist fractures, and certain diseases appear to predispose people to develop carpal tunnel syndrome. These diseases include diabetes and rheumatoid arthritis.

Diabetes is known to cause peripheral nerve damage, which can sensitize the nerves to compression and may make one more susceptible to carpal tunnel syndrome. Certain kinds of arthritis can cause the synovial tissue that lines the joints to become inflamed and swell. Because this same synovial tissue covers the tendons in the carpal tunnel, these types of arthritis may cause swelling in the carpal tunnel that may then cause compression of the median nerve and hence carpal tunnel syndrome. Kidney and heart problems can also result in swelling in the body, including the carpal tunnel, and can cause carpal tunnel syndrome. Finally, any type of growth or swelling in the carpal tunnel can also pinch the nerve and cause carpal tunnel syndrome.

Researchers have found that if electrical tests of the median nerve are performed on large numbers of people, some of those people may have slowing of nerve conduction but no symptoms of carpal tunnel syndrome. They may be at an increased risk of developing the condition, but more research needs to be done on this question.

By my definition, such individuals don't have carpal tunnel syndrome, although they may be at higher risk of developing it. I believe that the brain is much more sensitive to slowing of the nerve than any electrical test can be, so if you aren't having symptoms, your median nerve is working fine for you.

28 Is carpal tunnel syndrome becoming more common?

There's certainly a public perception that carpal tunnel syndrome is on the increase, but it's hard to pin down the reality. The apparent increases could be due to several causes.

For one thing, there could be a true increase in the syndrome itself. There is a perception that American workers are being asked to do more with their hands to increase productivity, but perhaps we're reaching the physiological limits of the body, and further increases in hand use will cause more cases of carpal tunnel syndrome.

Reported increases could also be due to more people with mild cases deciding to see their doctors. In addition, if doctors change their diagnostic criteria and make them more lenient, this would also cause an increase in the number of people diagnosed with the disease.

In other words, at this point it's hard to decide whether carpal tunnel syndrome is increasing or whether the statistics we hear about are the result of changes in how cases are defined and counted.

29 Is carpal tunnel syndrome a problem only in the United States?

Carpal tunnel syndrome occurs all over the world. It has received a lot of attention in the United States because of the controversy over repetitive strain injuries in the workplace. Part Four discusses these issues in more detail.

Interestingly, carpal tunnel syndrome was seen as a severe problem in Australia a couple of decades ago when it was linked with cumulative trauma disorders. At that time, the "epidemic" in the United States was in its infancy. An intense debate about the cause of the epidemic took place in the Australian medical literature. Were Americans dumping defective keyboards on unsuspecting Aussie workers? Was this an example of mass social hysteria? Were entrepreneurial medical experts feeding the frenzy? These are some of the thoughts that were publicly debated at the time. The truth was never clearly discovered because the laws governing workers' compensation were changed so that these injuries were no longer covered.

The disorder seems to be commonly diagnosed and treated in industrialized countries and does not seem to be as much of a problem in developing countries, but it's not clear whether this is related to priorities, causation, or some social phenomenon. The more developed industrialized countries usually have a workers' compensation system that compensates workers who are injured on the job. In countries where this does not exist, workers who develop physical problems and can't work may not get paid. So they may be far less likely to complain about hand or other symptoms. Alternatively, the fast pace and demands of production in industrialized societies may force workers to use their hands in ways that create symptoms that are not seen in less developed countries. The truth is simply not known.

30 *When was carpal tunnel syndrome first recognized, and when was the first carpal tunnel surgery performed?*

The gradual discovery that compression of the median nerve causes carpal tunnel syndrome is an interesting chapter in medical history.

In his 1988 article on the history and analysis of carpal tunnel syndrome, California surgeon G. B. Pfeffer describes the first mention of the condition. In 1854, British surgeon Sir James Paget offered what appears to be the first description of a patient with carpal tunnel syndrome. The patient had such severe numbness of the fingers that he developed ulcerations of the tips of the fingers from lack of feeling. Minor injuries that would typically heal with no problems left non-healing sores on the tips of his fingers. The patient had experienced a previous fracture at the distal end of the radius, an injury that we now know predisposes people to carpal tunnel syndrome.

Pfeffer also wrote that in 1880 Boston neurologist James Putnam clearly described carpal tunnel syndrome. And in the early 1900s, anatomists carrying out dissections of the hand noted that people with atrophy of the ball of the thumb also exhibited an hourglass-shaped narrowing, or deformity, of the median nerve in the carpal tunnel.

At first, most surgeons believed that nerve compression was located in the thoracic outlet (see Question 19) rather than in the carpal tunnel, but numerous attempts to cure the nerve compression surgically failed to relieve the symptoms. It wasn't until 1947 that a prominent English neurologist pointed out that compression of the median nerve in the carpal tunnel could explain the symptoms and physical findings of carpal tunnel syndrome.

At that point, surgeons began paying serious attention to the condition, and in 1947 George S. Phalen, the sixteenth president of the American Society for Surgery of the Hand, wrote that he made his first diagnosis of carpal tunnel syndrome. He later went on to write many influential articles about carpal tunnel syndrome that alerted the surgical community to the disorder, its symptoms, its physical findings, and its treatment.

Herbert Galloway, a Canadian orthopedic surgeon in Winnipeg, Manitoba, Canada, performed the first carpal tunnel release in 1924 on a woman patient who had developed thumb and index finger problems and wasting of the ball of the thumb after a heavy object fell across the back of her wrist. The surgery gave her improved feeling in the fingers, but she developed pain in the scar. Galloway operated on her a second time, but the repeat surgery failed to give her complete relief from her symptoms.

The next published report of carpal tunnel surgery was carried out at the Mayo Clinic in 1933. Research at the clinic also played a central role in advancing understanding of nerve compression and carpal tunnel syndrome, with J. R. Learmonth, M.D., performing some of the earliest surgery.

Despite the clear descriptions of the symptoms dating back decades, however, by 1950 only twelve patients had undergone surgical release of the carpal tunnel for what is now called idiopathic carpal tunnel syndrome.

At present, carpal tunnel release is the most common hand procedure carried out by U.S. hand surgeons, with an estimated 400,000 surgeries performed each year.

Endnotes for Question 30

PFEFFER, G. B., ET AL., "The History of Carpal Tunnel Surgery," *Journal of Hand Surgery* (British and European Volume, 1988), 13B, 1: 28–34. This article reviews the history of carpal tunnel syndrome. The authors believe there was a delay in understanding carpal tunnel syndrome because powerful surgeons were interested in competing explanations of symptoms.

PHALEN, GEORGE S., "The Carpal-Tunnel Syndrome: Seventeen Years' Experience in Diagnosis and Treatment of Six Hundred Fifty-Four Hands," *The Journal of Bone and Joint Surgery,* 48A, no. 2 (March 1966): 211–227. This is a landmark paper about carpal tunnel syndrome that formed the foundation for the evaluation and care of patients with this condition. It remains relevant today, and, because of its comprehensive nature, is a useful reference regarding the status of carpal tunnel syndrome in the 1960s.

AMADIO, P. C., "The First Carpal Tunnel Release," *Journal of Hand Surgery* (British and European Volume, 1995), 20B, 1: 40–41. This article recounts the first carpal tunnel surgery.

Part Four

Hands at Work:
Carpal Tunnel Syndrome, the Workplace, and the Repetitive Stress Injury Controversy

Introduction

Upper-extremity complaints—problems in the hands and arms—are probably second only to back pain as the biggest medical problems in industry today because thousands of workers are blaming their jobs for their medical difficulties. Whether workplace environments and activities are actually causing conditions such as carpal tunnel syndrome is one of the major questions that hand surgeons are trying to answer. The problem is that it may not be answerable, at least not without much more research.

It's only human nature to want to know the cause of any problem that arises. We're creatures who want answers and causes, so naturally, because so many millions of us spend at least eight hours a day, five days a week, at work, we tend to attribute symptoms, discomfort, or pain to the workplace. But most health problems, like many aspects of human existence, are caused by a combination of factors acting in concert, and it may be impossible to figure out the main cause, or even assess how the various causes are interacting to create the condition.

For example, I once had to testify in a workers' compensation case regarding a patient who had both carpal tunnel syndrome and diabetes. When I was asked to state how much of the numbness was caused by the diabetes and how much was caused by the workplace, I could only reply, "It's impossible to estimate." The lawyers looked at me in disbelief. They were trying to force a cause into existence, but in my view the two causes were inseparable. The patient might never have had numbness if he hadn't had diabetes, and he might never have had numbness if he hadn't entered his particular occupation.

In Western medicine, the standard procedure for trying to develop a link between a condition and its causes is to conduct research. When seeking the causes of carpal tunnel syndrome, for example, we would take people with the condition and people who don't have it and ask them about their activities, including using computer keyboards and other repetitive activities. Over time, and with enough research, we may come up with satisfactory answers. If you believe that work is causing your condition, however, you're entitled to seek treatment for it, and if you've had a workplace injury that has resulted in a permanent impairment, you're entitled to receive compensation. This may take place in an atmosphere of confrontation, but it is still your right.

Why is the issue of workplace injury so often colored by confrontation? I believe that a great deal of the conflict is a kind of "illness" itself, caused by laws, regulations, and the competing economic interests that are reflected in laws and regulations. Diseases and health conditions are not independent entities but are also matters of social definition, and definitions can change over time. This is what I meant in the preface when I stated that carpal tunnel syndrome is a kind of symbol that reflects societal values and tensions. It takes place in a social context.

The truth is, you may not have it in your power to modify that social context, so the healthiest stance you can take is to be proactive in taking care of your health, accept the possibility that resolving workplace injuries may turn adversarial, develop good negotiating skills, deal with what you can, focus your energy on getting better, and enjoy everything that's good in your life. Both your physical and emotional well-being will benefit if you maintain a healthy, positive outlook.

31 Are there anatomical and physiological reasons for linking repetitive work activities and carpal tunnel syndrome?

Researchers into carpal tunnel syndrome have developed several theories to explain how repetitive work might cause carpal tunnel syndrome.

Interest initially focused on the lining of the flexor tendons, which, as described in Part Two, pass through the carpal tunnel and connect the muscles in the forearm to the fingers. You can feel your own forearm muscles flex when you make a tight fist. A loose supportive tissue called *synovium* or *synovial tissue* lines the flexor tendons in the carpal tunnel. In certain medical conditions such as rheumatoid arthritis, disease can cause inflammation and swelling in the synovium, resulting in carpal tunnel syndrome. This has made surgeons suspect that swelling in the synovium might be a cause of carpal tunnel syndrome that could be worsened by vigorous gripping. Pressure measurements taken after gripping show increased pressure in the carpal tunnel, but biopsies of the synovium taken at the time of carpal tunnel release have not shown changes.

Muscles from above and below are close to the carpal tunnel and are suspected as a cause of carpal tunnel syndrome. Two large groups of muscles in the forearm are responsible for flexing the fingers. The superficial group, called the *flexor digitorum superficialis* ("superficial finger flexors") lies very close to the carpal tunnel and forms tendons in the forearm just above the carpal tunnel. These tendons traverse the tunnel, and, in some people, the superficial finger flexor muscles can actually lie in the carpal tunnel when the fingers are straightened.

We know that muscles get larger with exercise and that repetitive work is in fact a form of exercise for the muscles. So it seems logical that some people who perform repetitive work and have flexor muscles that encroach on the carpal tunnel might be more prone to develop carpal tunnel syndrome; in this case, the condition could be work related.

A corollary to this theory is that the flexor muscles seem to encroach more on the carpal tunnel in short people, an interesting point if you recall that women are usually shorter than men and that carpal tunnel syndrome is more common in women.

Muscles from the hand are also of interest as possible culprits in causing carpal tunnel syndrome. In our palms are small, thin muscles that connect the tendons that flex and extend the fingers. To the anatomist who named them centuries ago, these muscles looked a bit like worms and thus they were called *lumbricals,* which means "earth-worm" in Latin. These muscles are unusual because they join one tendon to another rather than joining a tendon to a bone. In any case, the lumbricals regulate the balance between the flexor tendons and the extensor tendons. When the flexor muscles grip, the lumbricals relax and let the finger bend. When the finger straightens, they pull on the flexor muscles, stretching them so there will be less resistance to straightening the finger.

In someone with large flexor muscles, for example, someone who performs a repetitive gripping job, the lumbricals will receive a great deal of exercise and may grow. Researchers have in fact discovered, based on anatomic dissection and magnetic resonance imaging (MRI) scans, that the lumbricals can encroach on the distal end of the carpal tunnel and may pinch the nerve.

Finally, recent research using ultrasound has shown that the median nerve itself actually enlarges after vigorous activity.

32 Is my work causing my carpal tunnel syndrome, and should I claim it as a work-related injury?

As suggested in the introduction to this section, there are no easy answers to these questions.

It's obvious that certain hand positions increase pressure in the carpal tunnel. If your work demands that you hold your wrist in a highly flexed or extended position for prolonged periods of time and your hand becomes numb in the area covered by the median nerve while you are in this position, then it seems likely that your carpal tunnel syndrome is due at least in part to your work. In recent years, many jobs that require constant wrist flexion or extension have been modified.

The possible relationship between carpal tunnel syndrome and work that requires repetitive gripping, such as the use of pistol-grip power guns to drive screws or tighten bolts in modern manufacturing, is less clear. Scientific research is not conclusive on this point, but most surgeons and insurance carriers believe that these kinds of activities may aggravate carpal tunnel syndrome and cause symptoms to worsen.

The relationship between keyboarding and carpal tunnel syndrome is even muddier. The number of workers' compensation claims for carpal tunnel syndrome as a result of keyboard use have certainly multiplied over the past ten years, but whether this activity can actually cause the condition is a research issue that may take years to resolve.

If you experience symptoms primarily at night but not at your workplace, it seems less likely that your work is causing your condition. If your symptoms come on while you're at work, then it's possible that your work activities are at least exacerbating your carpal tunnel syndrome.

Carpal tunnel syndrome rarely develops due to one specific event. It more typically comes on gradually over time. The legal regulations for attributing a condition to the workplace vary from country to country and in different regions of the United States. This indicates that at this point in history, attributing carpal tunnel syndrome to the workplace is more an administrative decision than a medical one, so I'd recommend that you become informed about the regulations for workplace attribution in your own state.

If you feel that your work is causing your medical condition, your company will generally ask you to file a claim. This will usually trigger a visit to a doctor for a diagnosis, treatment recommendations, and quite possibly an opinion about whether the condition is work related.

If you have concerns about how your work may be affecting your overall musculoskeletal health, Part Nine contains some very effective exercises and suggestions for protecting yourself from developing carpal tunnel syndrome, and possibly other conditions as well.

33 If I go to a doctor for an employment-related condition, will the doctor be working for me or for the insurance company?

Most doctors will try to provide you with the very best evaluation and treatment for your condition, but doctors who have created a niche in workers' compensation may make decisions and diagnoses based on the cost to the insurance carrier and your employer. You'll be able to identify them by how they treat you. Their first strategy will be to deny that a condition is related to the workplace. Second, they will not recommend surgical treatment, and if surgery is performed, they will try to return you to work early—although this is a stance I tend to agree with because returning to work disrupts your life less, minimizes the "disabled patient" mind-set that arises with inactivity, and helps to promote the physical healing process. Finally, when the time comes to calculate a permanent impairment, they will tend to lowball the rating used to calculate your financial settlement.

As an informed patient, you should be aware that these types of physicians exist. Your fellow employees will no doubt know their names. Feel free to ask for a second opinion at any time in the course of your treatment for any condition. If a second opinion is required before surgery, for example, always ask if you have the right to choose the doctor who will provide that second opinion. If you can't choose the doctor for the second opinion, seek a third opinion on your own, and be willing to pay for it out of your own pocket if necessary. In some states, patients have the right to choose their own doctors in a workers' compensation case. In others, the employer has the right to choose the doctor who will examine an injured worker. Whatever rules apply in your state, it's worthwhile to inform yourself about how the system works.

If you end up with three opinions that are all the same, you should probably accept that the advice is appropriate for your condition. In other words, don't embark on a quest for an opinion that will reinforce what you want to believe.

34 What's the difference between an "impairment rating" and a "disability rating"?

A "rating" or an "impairment rating" identifies the impairment that has been left in your hand or body after an injury or illness. It's the most common method used to identify the permanent effects of an injury and is the basis on which a financial settlement is calculated if you've been injured at work.

If you've experienced a workplace injury, undergone treatment, and improved to the fullest extent possible, you've recovered to what is called your Maximum Medical Improvement (MMI). When patients are at MMI, they aren't expected to get any better, nor are they expected to have further active medical testing or treatment.

When you reach MMI, the insurance carrier will ask your doctor to determine whether you have any permanent physical effects or body defects as a result of the injury. These permanent effects are called "impairments," physical defects that the doctor can measure. Your doctor creates an impairment rating by comparing your condition to the *American Medical Association's Impairment Manual*. The workers' compensation insurance carrier uses this rating, along with a formula, to calculate the financial settlement you'll receive.

"Disability" refers to limitations that you may be subject to in your day-to-day activities because of the impairment. For example, if you lose the tip of your little finger, you might have an impairment of 2 percent of your entire body, but you may not be disabled. You could possibly still do everything. If you were a professional violinist, however, and suffered the same injury, your impairment would still be 2 percent but you would probably be 100 percent disabled from your work. Doctors usually measure impairments and provide you and your insurance carrier with an impairment rating, but patients often ask for "disability ratings" because of confusion in the terminology.

You owe it to yourself to read everything you receive and make sure you understand everything you are asked to sign about your impairment, your disability, and your settlement.

35 My earlier carpal tunnel syndrome was covered by a workers' compensation claim. Now it has come back. Is it still covered?

Regulations for workers' compensation vary widely from state to state. You should protect yourself by becoming informed about the regulations in your state before you sign anything or agree to any long-term settlement.

Many hand surgery practices have nurses who are experienced in and knowledgeable about the workers' compensation regulations in their states. In some states, new symptoms attributed to an old claim will be covered under that claim.

36 What are the implications of defining carpal tunnel syndrome as a work-related condition?

Although regulations vary from state to state, employees who suffer an injury at work usually receive medical care for that problem. If they lose time from work, they usually receive some type of salary replacement. Finally, if they experience a permanent change or disability as a result of a work-related injury, they may receive financial compensation for the loss.

If the injury is in truth attributable to the workplace, most of us would see this as a fair and reasonable course of events. Unfortunately, with carpal tunnel syndrome, two potential problems can occur. First, the diagnosis can be in doubt; second, the workplace may not be the cause of the carpal tunnel syndrome. This introduces uncertainty into the situation.

Because there may be financial implications for both the employee and the employer, each will champion his or her own perspective.

This can lead to an adversarial relationship between employee and employer that may have negative consequences.

If a worker isn't "bleeding on the floor," the more cynical people at the workplace may doubt the presence of any condition at all. If the complaining employee asks for and is given modified tasks, others who are working hard and who may have symptoms of their own will feel that the individual is getting a "sweet deal" and taking advantage of the employer and fellow workers. They may ostracize the injured worker. The employer may believe that the employee has nothing wrong with him or her and feel trapped or exploited by the circumstances. Regulations governing the safety of the work environment may force the employer to provide modified tasks or even make an expensive investment in unproven and possibly faddish ergonomic interventions.

So, as you can see, although the medical condition of carpal tunnel syndrome is the same in working and nonworking populations, a case of carpal tunnel syndrome that is defined as work related can have a lot of implications.

37 Is there any difference between a repetitive strain injury and a cumulative trauma disorder?

Repetitive strain injury (RSI) and *cumulative trauma disorder (CTD)* both refer to the same concept. Some physicians and researchers believe that when tissues are used in a forceful, repetitive fashion, the continuous process of tissue repair and rejuvenation can become overwhelmed. If the microinjuries caused by these activities are not given the rest time required for normal tissue repair, the injuries may accumulate and eventually cause symptoms such as pain and difficulties in using the hand and arm.

This is a controversial area because some doctors doubt the very existence of these problems. RSI and CTD are also the subject of much discussion, not just in medicine but also in industry, in insurance circles, and among policymakers.

38 Do you believe that carpal tunnel syndrome is due to repetitive stress or cumulative trauma?

Carpal tunnel syndrome is often considered an RSI or CTD, but there is no widely accepted proof that it is in fact the result of cumulative trauma.

I find the theory of cumulative trauma logical, but I'm not convinced that cumulative microtrauma leads to pressure on the median nerve. I believe that other anatomic theories, such as those discussed at the beginning of this section, are much more attractive as a cause of the current epidemic of carpal tunnel syndrome.

For one thing, we don't know yet whether RSIs and CTDs really exist. Carpal tunnel syndrome is an accepted disorder caused by pressure on the median nerve in the carpal tunnel. It doesn't share the features of other cumulative trauma disorders in that no actual tissue injury is needed to cause carpal tunnel syndrome, nor is any actual injury needed to increase pressure on the nerve.

By linking carpal tunnel syndrome to a group of disorders that are controversial and poorly understood, we are assuming the existence of RSIs or CTDs when there may be no such physical entity. This clouds the picture for carpal tunnel syndrome.

For example, repetitive gripping may cause carpal tunnel syndrome, but enough anatomic possibilities exist to explain this connection without inventing an entirely new disease process of cumulative microinjury. We may not know enough about disease to explain other upper-limb conditions, but carpal tunnel syndrome fits well into our current thinking about nerve compression.

It's possible that CTDs are simply a way for a doctor to say, "I don't know what's causing this condition." As humans, we have a strong need to put labels on things because we think that helps us to understand them. But labeling may also create something that doesn't yet exist in a real way, and this may be the case for CTDs.

39 *Why do people believe that RSIs and CTDs exist?*

In Western medicine, we judge theories by evidence. A new theory of disease such as RSI and CTD must explain not only what is known and understood by earlier theories but must also explain what has been observed but not explained by those earlier theories.

Because we appear to be facing clinical entities that are different and do not behave like what we've seen and been able to explain in the past, a new theory of what is happening with repetitive work may be useful. Several pieces of evidence tell us that something is going on.

First, many people are coming to their doctors complaining of similar symptoms. Maybe this is a social phenomenon; however, the symptoms are complex, and I find it hard to believe that all these patients could develop similar symptoms just from reading reports in newspapers or magazines.

The existing theories of nerve compression and physical injury that we relied on before the concept of RSIs and CTDs emerged don't explain this new group of patients, whose conditions are difficult to diagnose and treat. Are these patients suffering from some combination of physical and emotional disorders that has been created by social issues in the workplace rather than by an actual disease? Maybe, but we don't yet have a cohesive theory that would explain these observations in a way that health-care professionals and researchers accept.

Second, research has shown a relationship between force and repetitiveness of work activities and the existence of upper-limb symptoms.

Third, the existing models for explaining disease and injury don't clarify our current clinical observations.

And fourth, a new disease entity called CTD or RSI could explain more of these observations.

If this theory is going to be helpful, we must be able to test it. How can we do this? One method is to predict ways of treating the disorder, for example, with rest, and then to see if these treatments cure the condition. This has been done to some extent, but patients with RSIs and CTDs often fail to get better with rest. Patients can continue to suffer from symptoms for years after they have been forced to stop working.

Furthermore, we have seen no convincing signs of tissue injury when we carry out microscopic tissue evaluations in RSI patients. And although patients may continue to have severe symptoms over time, they don't develop purely objective signs of disease as the problem progresses.

All these factors fail to prove the existence of RSIs and make them one of the greatest medical mysteries of our time. Still, although we have no proof that RSIs and CTDs exist, we can't deny that something is happening in society that will someday teach us a great deal about the relationships among the hand, the mind, and the workplace.

Part Five

Getting Help:
How Doctors Diagnose and
Treat Carpal Tunnel Syndrome

Introduction

When you decide to visit a doctor about your symptoms, he or she will try to determine their cause and how they can be relieved. Some of the questions and tests will help determine what is wrong with your hand, some may help the doctor estimate the severity of your problem, and some are designed to help decide what type of treatment could be most beneficial.

Medical diagnosis and treatment are complex processes, and you'll stand the best chance of getting help if you are completely honest. Patients should never feel that they're under any obligation to please their doctors or to tell them what they think the doctors might want to hear. Your doctor will try her best to help you get better, and if you conceal your concerns or don't mention aspects of your condition because they frighten you, or because you feel that the doctor should be able to guess what's wrong, you make her task much harder and reduce your chances of being helped.

When trying to figure out what's wrong with you, your doctor must examine you, which means touching you. If you feel uneasy about being touched, try to think about what will make you feel more comfortable, and ask the doctor to go along with your wishes. In examinations that involve anything of a personal nature, such as gynecological exams, a third person usually stays in the room at all times. For hand examinations, most doctors leave the door of the examining room open. Your doctor should explain everything to you before the examination or as it proceeds, and if you feel at all uncomfortable, ask whatever questions you may have.

After the examination, your doctor may recommend further tests. There are several reasons for tests. Your doctor may suspect that you have a certain condition but does not have enough evidence to "nail it down." If the treatment for the condition has possible negative side effects, if it's dangerous, or even if it's costly, your doctor may want to be as sure as possible that you have that condition before recommending that treatment. Other reasons might be to evaluate how severe your condition is or to see if treatment is having a positive effect.

When you become a patient, you give up some control over your life. But you're always in the driver's seat. When it comes to hand problems, it's your hand, and it's your right to have a say in how it is treated.

This is rather like hiring an expert to inspect a house that I am planning to buy. I'd let the inspector carry out the inspection and give me a report, and then I'd ask questions about any parts of the report that I didn't understand or that really mattered to me. I would get the inspector's advice about the house, but it would still be up to me to buy the house or not.

Similarly, it's your doctor's job to tell you what he believes is the nature of your problem, to give you the results of examinations and tests, and to recommend treatment, but it's your decision whether to go along with those recommendations. These are very personal choices, and only you, the patient, can make them. You also always have the option of getting second or third opinions. Even if your insurance doesn't cover this, you can pay for it yourself.

40 If I have had symptoms, how long should I wait before going to see a doctor?

It's hard to give exact advice about when you should see a doctor about hand symptoms.

If you're having a symptom such as numbness that doesn't go away or seems to be getting worse or more frequent, you should check with a doctor. You should also have an evaluation if you have symptoms that cause you discomfort or interfere with your being able to use your hands. If you've developed a new symptom—something you haven't experienced before—you should have it investigated. Finally, if you're being treated for carpal tunnel syndrome and your symptoms fail to improve, you should go back for another checkup.

41 Can my family doctor or primary care physician evaluate and treat my carpal tunnel syndrome?

When nerve compression may be involved, it's important to come up with an accurate diagnosis and to rule out other possible causes of symptoms.

I believe that family doctors and primary care physicians are an excellent place to start for any health concern. They are qualified to carry out the initial examination, evaluation, and diagnosis, and can begin treating you for carpal tunnel syndrome. Because you've had a relationship in the past, your family doctor is in the best position to provide initial evaluations and to provide most of your health-care needs.

Both family doctors and primary care doctors are at the front line for most health problems. Family doctors receive training in a wide range of areas, including children's care, reproductive issues, care of the aging, and counseling, and also undergo a special residency or apprenticeship specific to the family practice environment. Family doctors will treat your entire family and will make appropriate referrals when needed.

Primary care doctors have the training and experience to treat individual patients but may specialize in caring for certain population groups. For example, pediatricians are primary care doctors for children, but they wouldn't treat the elderly. Primary care doctors are often family doctors, specialists in internal medicine, pediatricians, or sometimes obstetrician/gynecologists.

42 How will my doctor decide whether I really have carpal tunnel syndrome?

Doctors are able to decide with a high degree of certainty whether a person has carpal tunnel syndrome by evaluating her symptoms and carrying out a physical examination. First, we'll ask you questions about your symptoms as part of your medical history, which is the most important method of gathering information about your health. Then we'll perform a physical examination appropriate for your symptoms.

Putting together the information from your medical history and the physical examination will, in most cases, allow us to make a diagnosis—in other words, put a name to your condition. Based on the diagnosis, we'll then suggest treatment possibilities, because any condition may be treated in a variety of ways.

The medical history usually contains a strong suggestion of nerve compression. By the time you've given your history, we'll have a good idea of whether you have carpal tunnel syndrome. In the physical examination, we try to confirm whether nerve compression is causing your symptoms and where the nerve is compressed. We also try to measure the severity of compression and evaluate you for other illnesses that could influence the diagnosis or your treatment.

The physical examination usually starts with a simple inspection of your hands and arms. We gain a great deal of information—the strength of your muscles, the appearance of calluses, whether you bite your nails—just by looking. Then we palpate, or feel, your hands and arms to determine whether there are any swellings on the nerve or if the nerves are tender at any specific location.

Provocative tests are physical examination maneuvers that are used to provoke symptoms. Because the compressed nerve is sensitive, tests that cause it to be compressed further can provoke symptoms. Some of the provocative tests used to diagnose carpal tunnel syndrome are discussed later in this section. We also measure the function of the nerve, using specific tests for sensory and motor functions. Finally, we put all this information together and come up with recommendations for further testing or treatment.

Sometimes, we aren't quite sure of the diagnosis. Where possible carpal tunnel syndrome is involved, we may recommend further tests, described in the questions that follow.

43 How will my doctor determine the severity of my carpal tunnel syndrome?

If your symptoms are recent, intermittent, not too bothersome, and come on with specific postures or at night, your diagnosis might be mild carpal tunnel syndrome. At this stage, your physical examination may be completely normal.

If your symptoms have gotten worse—becoming more frequent and severe, and perhaps coming on with less provocation—you may have moderate carpal tunnel syndrome. At this stage, the physical examination and tests may be positive, making it easier to make an accurate diagnosis.

Finally, the symptoms of severe carpal tunnel syndrome include continuous or almost continuous hand numbness, shrinking or wasting of the *thenar* muscle (see Question 48 and Figure 9) at the ball of the thumb, and a decrease in your normal ability to feel things and to discriminate between one and two points touching your skin.

Other tests, such as electrical testing of the median nerve discussed later in this section, provide information about the severity of your condition.

44 What kinds of tests are used to diagnose carpal tunnel syndrome?

As indicated previously, we have a wide range of tests, performed in the office and in the laboratory, to diagnose carpal tunnel syndrome. Among those that your doctor will carry out during your physical examination are Phalen's test, the provocative pressure test, and Tinel's sign, discussed later. These are all designed to detect nerve compression in your neck, arm, carpal tunnel, or other areas. These are commonly termed *provocative tests* because they attempt to induce or "provoke" the numbness and pain that are symptoms of nerve compression.

If your median nerve is compressed, and your doctor compresses it further by positioning your hand and arm in a specific manner, as in Phalen's test, or by compressing the nerve externally, as in the provocative pressure test, symptoms of nerve compression will appear if you have carpal tunnel syndrome. These tests are used to confirm the location where the nerve is compressed.

Other tests, such as the two-point discrimination test and muscle strength testing, determine how severely the nerve is compressed by evaluating its sensory and motor functions.

Finally, your doctor may choose from a range of additional tests to determine whether other conditions might be causing your symptoms or if you have other medical conditions that could affect either the treatment of your carpal tunnel syndrome or your chances for recovery.

45 What is Phalen's test?

Phalen's test is named for hand surgeon George S. Phalen, mentioned in Part Three. He was instrumental in teaching the hand surgery community about carpal tunnel syndrome in the 1950s and 1960s, and he invented this simple physical examination test.

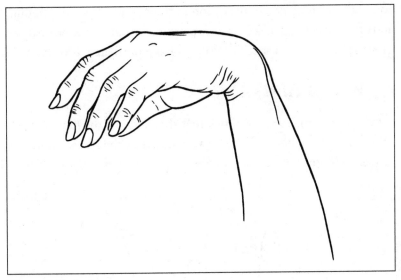

Figure 7. Phalen's test

Your doctor will ask you to flex your wrists toward the inside of your forearm to a 90-degree angle for one minute (see Figure 7). Most people with carpal tunnel syndrome (and some who don't have it) will develop numbness in the fingers served by the median nerve within one minute of assuming this posture. This result is generally viewed as a positive finding for carpal tunnel syndrome.

The thinking behind this test is straightforward, for if your nerve is already marginally compressed, the increased pressure on the nerve caused by flexing the wrist will provoke the symptoms of numbness. In fact, this may be the nighttime posture that brings on numbness of the hands during sleep.

46 *What is the provocative pressure test?*

In the provocative pressure test (see Figure 8), your doctor presses his or her thumb directly over the median nerve at the carpal tunnel or at other areas where nerve compression is suspected. If you feel numbness in your hand within one minute of compression, this is a positive finding and offers evidence that you have carpal tunnel syndrome or nerve compression, either at that specific location or at more than one location.

47 What is Tinel's sign?

Tinel's sign is an electrical shock that shoots down the hand, or any other part of the body, in the area governed by the nerve when it is tapped. The tingling sensation you feel when you hit your "funny

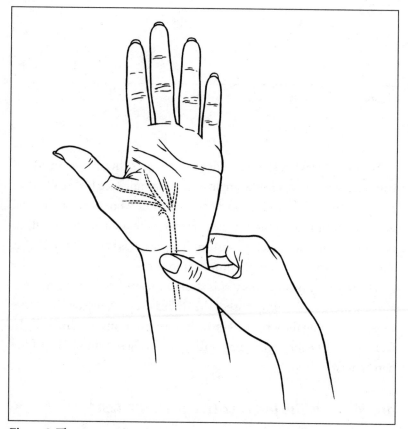

Figure 8. The provocative pressure test

bone" is a Tinel's sign of the ulnar nerve under the elbow. A positive Tinel's sign is evidence of an irritated nerve and can help localize the site of nerve compression.

48 How will my doctor measure the severity of my nerve compression?

The severity of nerve compression is tested by checking how sensitive the hand is to stimuli. One common test is the two-point discrimination test, which measures your ability to distinguish whether one or two points are touching the skin of your hand. When evaluating the major nerves of the arm and hand, it's usually performed on the pulp of the fingers.

Most hand surgeons use the tips of an open paper clip to touch the hand at two points a couple of millimeters apart (you can try this at home). If your median and ulnar nerves are functioning normally, you'll have no trouble discriminating the sensation of one point from two, even if the two points are only a few millimeters apart.

In severe nerve compression, you'll lose the ability to distinguish two points. This ability also diminishes naturally to some extent with age or if you have thick calluses on your fingers.

Your doctor will also test the motor component of the median nerve by observing and measuring the strength of the *thenar* muscles of the ball of the thumb. To do this, you lay your hand flat on a table, palm up, then lift your thumb to the ceiling. Your doctor will test and record the strength of this movement. In cases of severe or long-standing carpal tunnel syndrome, the thenar muscle, which is served by the median nerve, may shrink or atrophy (see Figure 9), and there may be weakness on testing. Weakness in other muscles of the hand and arm is not associated with or caused by carpal tunnel syndrome. Doctors usually recommend carpal tunnel surgery if the compression is so severe that the thenar muscles have atrophied.

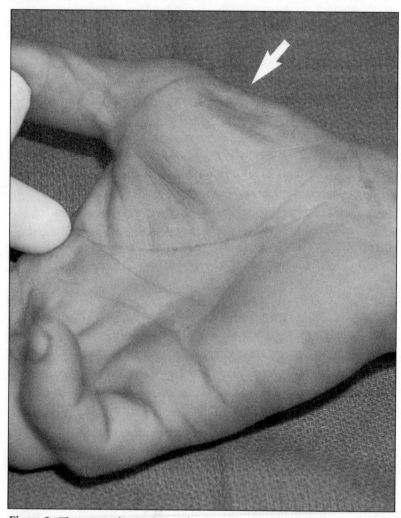

Figure 9. Thenar muscle atrophy

49 *Are x-rays, CAT scans, and MRI useful in diagnosing carpal tunnel syndrome?*

In x-rays, a beam of radiation is passed through body tissues and recorded on a photographic plate. The denser the tissue, the more of the x-ray beam will be blocked. The lungs, which contain air, stop very few of the x-rays, whereas bones stop much more. If a bone is fractured, the x-rays pass through the fracture but are blocked by the neighboring bone, thus recording a picture of the fracture on film. When the photographic plate is developed, it gives a picture of the body part that was x-rayed. Doctors can interpret the image and use the information it offers to make diagnoses and to decide on treatments.

Tomograms are an advanced form of x-ray in which the film and machine move over the patient or the body part while a series of x-rays is taken. Most of the picture is blurred, but certain parts of the body can be focused on in great detail, and putting several tomograms together creates a three-dimensional image. CT or CAT scans refer to the process of connecting tomograms to a computer for analysis.

Because the median nerve, like other nerves, is soft tissue and much less dense than bones, it doesn't show up on regular x-rays. However, x-rays will reveal problems with the carpal bones that can cause swelling in the region and thus carpal tunnel syndrome. So they're useful for revealing these problems and helpful when it comes time to plan treatment for the underlying cause of the patient's carpal tunnel syndrome.

As mentioned, distal radius fracture, the most common wrist fracture, is a known cause of carpal tunnel syndrome. With the help of x-rays that show how the fracture healed, doctors can better define the cause and plan treatment for carpal tunnel symptoms.

In Question 21, which focused on arthritis of the neck, I mentioned MRI, or the magnetic resonance imaging technique that takes pictures of the inside of the body without using x-rays. Instead, the body part of interest is placed in a powerful magnet that affects the movement of the body's molecules. Depending on their makeup, body tissues respond differently to this magnetic field. These differences can be recorded and reconstructed to form a detailed image of the body.

Unlike x-rays, MRI can provide clear images of the median nerve, so this technology may allow much more accurate visualization of the nerve in the future. At the current time, the images obtained aren't clear enough and don't offer sufficient information to use MRI in routine decision making about the treatment of carpal tunnel syndrome.

MRI is excellent for locating swellings and tumors in the carpal tunnel, however, and can identify many types of pathology in the wrist and carpal tunnel region. As the price of this technology comes down, the images improve, and our experience with MRI grows, I predict that sooner or later MRI will become a standard diagnostic tool for all patients who complain of hand numbness and pain.

50 Is ultrasound useful in diagnosing carpal tunnel syndrome?

Ultrasound works by beaming a high-frequency sound wave into body tissues and measuring it as it rebounds. The sound wave passes through fluid and bounces off denser tissues, and the reflected sound is used to create an image of the underlying tissue. Ultrasound is the technology employed to take pictures of fetuses to estimate their age in the womb. It has increasing uses in obstetrics, gynecology, and abdominal surgery, and is used to study tissues such as the thyroid gland.

Many researchers are interested in exploring ultrasound imaging of the carpal tunnel and median nerve because it can provide a reasonably good picture of the area. It's increasingly being used to identify some of the causes of carpal tunnel syndrome but has not yet found its way into widespread clinical practice. As we gain more experience with this technique, we may find that ultrasound images of the median nerve and carpal tunnel will help us plan and follow up on treatment. At present, however, patients' symptoms and the physical examination are the most important pieces of information used to manage treatment.

51 *My doctor has recommended "nerve tests." What do they involve, and what will we learn from them?*

Nerve testing, also called *electrodiagnostic testing*, is the general term used to describe the process of measuring the electrical activity of the nerves to determine whether they display any of the characteristic changes associated with nerve compression or other nerve or muscle diseases.

Electrical testing for diagnosing carpal tunnel syndrome and its severity has two components. One measures nerve conduction velocity (NCV), and the other, the *electromyogram (EMG),* measures the electrical activity of the muscles. In the EMG, small sterile needle electrodes are inserted into the muscles to measure their electrical activity.

We know that if the nerve is compressed, its velocity or speed of conduction slows down. The NCV measures how fast the nerve conducts a signal between two electrodes by stimulating the nerve at one location and recording the electrical signal at a distant location. We measure conduction speed for both the sensory and the motor parts of the median nerve and then compare them to similar measurements for the ulnar nerve. The speed of conduction is measured as distance divided by time, usually meters per second, and is referred to as *latency,* because it tells us how long it takes for stimulation to travel a specific distance.

The EMG shows a characteristic pattern of electrical activity of the muscles in cases of severe nerve compression. When a healthy nerve is innervating a healthy muscle, the nerve stimulates electrical activity in the muscle by sending a biological message that passes electrical signals to the muscle, which then contracts. If a nerve is compressed, damaged, or cut, and no electrical signals are traveling along it to the muscle, the muscle will generate very little electrical activity on its own. However, it will be seeking a signal and will increase its receptiveness to biochemical transmitters, which circulate in the blood. The muscle will become so reactive that a tiny level of circulating transmitter will cause it to be electrically active, and the muscle will show signs of activity although it isn't receiving any signals from the nerve.

This motion, called *fibrillation,* is like the movement of a cluster of worms wriggling in a can. In cases of severe nerve compression, the needle electrodes detect the muscle's excitability and spontaneous movements and record a characteristic pattern.

Electrodiagnostic testing requires the use of an electrical stimulus to stimulate the nerve. This is a polite way of saying that you'll feel an electric shock that stimulates the nerve and travels down to your hand. This isn't fun, and some people find it very uncomfortable. Also, the EMG uses small needle electrodes that are inserted into the small muscles of your hand to measure their electrical activity. Once again, this is somewhat uncomfortable. If you're afraid of needles, tell your doctor or the technician before the test. These tests aren't dangerous, and a few kind words of reassurance will probably go a long way to ease your concern.

52 Must I have nerve tests before I start treatment for carpal tunnel syndrome?

The main reason to undergo electrical testing is if your doctor suspects something other than carpal tunnel syndrome; however, this condition can usually be diagnosed adequately based on your medical history and physical examination. Electrical testing increases the level of certainty that you truly have carpal tunnel syndrome, but most diagnoses are clear enough that testing isn't necessary before starting treatment.

If surgery appears appropriate, however, your doctor and your surgeon may request electrical testing to confirm the diagnosis and determine its severity. In addition, many surgeons require electrical testing before performing surgery.

53 What's the best treatment for carpal tunnel syndrome, and what will my doctor recommend first?

I wish I could tell you that there's one best treatment for carpal tunnel syndrome, but there isn't. However, we do have a range of treatments for reducing symptoms by reducing the pressure on the median nerve. These include nighttime splinting, which prevents you from assuming a posture that will compress the nerve at night; changing your activities, which can often be difficult to achieve; injections of steroid medications; or one of several types of surgical procedures. All of these treatments are designed to reduce the pressure on the median nerve.

Most doctors will recommend that you start by using a splint at night to see if it will relieve your symptoms. Splints are worn on the wrist to keep it straight at night. They don't have to be tight; their primary job is to keep the wrist from flexing to any great degree. Remember, your wrist position while you're sleeping can cause pressure on the median nerve, and by the time the hand and finger numbness wakes you up, the nerve is compressed. Often the first improvement that patients notice when they begin wearing splints at night is an improvement in their sleep. If you manage to prevent significant nerve compression during sleep, the nerve may recover on its own.

54 What is a splint, and where can I get one?

A splint used to treat carpal tunnel syndrome is a type of canvas and elastic sleeve that holds your wrist in a neutral position and keeps it from excessive flexion or extension at night and during any daytime activities that put pressure on the median nerve.

Because the splint maintains the carpal tunnel in its most unconstricted position, it gives the median nerve the maximum amount of space within the tunnel. Doctors often recommend specific kinds of splints based on the particular patient's condition. Your doctor may provide you with a splint, or you may get one from a physical therapist or orthotist, a specialist in custom-making appliances that support the body.

Actually, you can find splints adequate for treating carpal tunnel syndrome at many surgical supply stores and even at drugstores. When you look for a splint, be sure that it can hold your wrist in a neutral position, that it fits relatively loosely, and that you can sleep wearing it (see Question 56).

Many splints have flat metal strips built into them to prevent motion, but you may find that the bar irritates your palm, even if you wear the splint loosely; you'll have to judge this for yourself. Keep in mind that the wrist doesn't need to be completely immobile. Rather, the splint should fit comfortably while also preventing the wrist from excessive flexing or extending. If a splint is uncomfortable, you won't want to use it, and if you don't use it, it won't help you.

55 *How many hours a day should I wear my splint?*

It isn't a question of how many hours, but of relieving your symptoms. Most doctors usually start patients wearing splints only at night because pressure in the carpal tunnel is thought to increase at night due to the effects of gravity and also to pressure on the median nerve caused by the positions in which we sleep.

During the day, most people move their hands around a lot, so pressure in the carpal tunnel does not increase. If you find that specific activities cause your symptoms to worsen, you may find it helpful to wear the splint at those times. For example, if you feel tingling, buzzing, or numbness in your fingers and hand when you mop the floor, wear the splint when you're cleaning.

Similarly, if you have hand numbness that comes on while you drive, it might be helpful for you to wear your splint at that time. However, if wearing the splint interferes with your ability to handle the car, you must take safety issues into account. It's probably a good idea to check on this with your insurance carrier. Also, you might find that a different type of splint allows you to keep the wrist straight while not interfering with your ability to drive.

Even if you wear the splint during the day, it's important that you also keep it on at night when you're sleeping and not in control of your hand and arm movements.

56 *What should I do if the splint I bought at the drugstore is uncomfortable? What if I can't sleep wearing my splint?*

If you've given your off-the-shelf splint a fair try for a week or two but are still so uncomfortable that you can't sleep while wearing it, you should make an appointment to see your doctor and confirm the diagnosis of carpal tunnel syndrome.

At that time, your doctor can also give you a prescription for a custom-made wrist splint that will be fashioned specifically to fit your hand. Orthotists and hand therapists make these types of custom splints.

If you can't wear your splint comfortably at night, whether it's a drugstore one or a custom one, you'll stop wearing it and it won't help you. First, make sure that you aren't fastening it too tightly. You might also try putting it on a half-hour or an hour before you go to bed so that your hand gets used to it before you try to sleep.

My other suggestion is: stick with it and be patient. The first night, it'll probably feel uncomfortable, but the body adapts with remarkable speed. You'll probably find that your comfort level improves each night and that after three or four nights you'll probably forget that you're even wearing the splint.

57 *How can I tell if my splint is working?*

If your splint is working, your symptoms will start to improve. You may notice that you're sleeping better at night and that you're not waking up in the middle of the night with numbness. These improvements may begin after the first few nights of wearing your splint, or they may take place gradually, over several weeks, as controlling your wrist position keeps the nerve from becoming compressed at night. In many cases, the nerve will recover and your symptoms will resolve.

If a month of night splinting fails to lessen your symptoms, however, it's unlikely that this simple treatment is going to solve your problem. In that case, you should go back to your doctor for another checkup, further diagnosis, and other treatment options.

58 My doctor says that "injecting" my carpal tunnel is a good first treatment. What does this involve?

"Injecting" the carpal tunnel is a shorthand way of referring to injecting steroid medications such as cortisone, sometimes mixed with a local anesthetic such as novocaine, into the carpal tunnel to relieve the symptoms of carpal tunnel syndrome. It's a common technique that many doctors combine with splinting as a first treatment.

Injection is often effective in relieving the symptoms of carpal tunnel syndrome because it reduces inflammation, and thus the volume of synovial tissue that lines the flexor tendons in the carpal tunnel. Reducing the volume of the tissue increases the amount of space in the tunnel and apparently reduces pressure on the median nerve.

If your carpal tunnel syndrome is the result of an inflammatory process such as rheumatoid arthritis, the injection will reduce the inflammation and may give you dramatic relief.

59 How long do the effects of the injection last?

You may experience improvement within the first few days after the injection, or it may take a week or two to have an effect. If you don't experience any improvement with a combination of splinting and the injection within a few months of treatment, you and your doctor may have to consider surgery. Unfortunately, there aren't a lot of other options with the exception of changing your work or other activities that may be contributing to your condition; however, those kinds of changes may be much more disruptive to your life than surgery.

Sometimes one or two injections alleviate all the symptoms permanently and patients need no further treatment. In my experience, about 50 percent of patients who are treated with splinting and injection fall into this category.

Your doctor can repeat the injection if the first one fails to relieve your symptoms or if it gives you relief for a while but your symptoms recur. If two injections have not given you long-lasting relief, it's unlikely that this treatment will solve your problem, so your doctor may recommend electrodiagnostic testing, if you've not yet had that done or the diagnosis is not clear. If the testing indicates carpal tunnel syndrome, your doctor will probably recommend surgery.

60 Is the injection painful?

The injection may be uncomfortable, if not somewhat painful. After all, it involves inserting a needle into the skin of the wrist and into the carpal tunnel itself. But there are ways to minimize the discomfort.

When injecting the carpal tunnel, your doctor or the nurse will first wash the skin of your wrist with a disinfectant, usually an alcohol solution, to kill bacteria on the skin. Some doctors add a bit of local anesthetic to the cortisone. Others numb the skin in the wrist area with an initial injection of novocaine or another local anesthetic and follow that with the injection of the cortisone. Using the smallest needle possible and injecting the drugs slowly also go a long way to reduce any discomfort. With a local anesthetic, most patients will not find the injection terribly uncomfortable.

In some cases of carpal tunnel syndrome, the area around the nerve can be very sensitive, and injection may be more painful, but this happens very rarely.

61 What side effects, if any, are associated with injection?

Any medical procedure carries with it a slight chance of infection, but the incidence of infection following carpal tunnel injections is probably less than one in a thousand.

Very rarely, a patient will have an allergic reaction either to the steroid drug or to the local anesthetic. If you're going to react, it's likely to happen almost immediately following the injection while you're still in the doctor's office, so you will be able to receive any necessary care. If you're like most people, you'll have had local anesthetics administered in the past by your dentist. If you've ever had an allergic reaction to novocaine or to any other drug, be sure the information is in your medical chart. And even if all the relevant information is in your chart, it never hurts to remind your doctor or the medical technician or nurse administering the treatment about any allergies before you undergo treatment. Some medical practices have a policy of asking patients to sign a patient information and consent form before undergoing injection, but most of the time, since you're not going to be under an anesthetic, your consent is assumed when your doctor explains the injection and you agree to it.

One relatively common side effect of steroid drugs is a shrinkage in fat tissues at the injection site that can make the tendons and veins more visible under the skin. Steroids can also cause depigmentation of the skin at the injection site. However, these changes in fatty tissue and skin color are rare in carpal tunnel injection because the drug is usually injected beneath the subcutaneous fat, which lies just under the skin.

If you're concerned about newspaper articles that talk about steroids causing weight gain or excessive muscle growth, you should realize that the steroid medication used in these injections is locally active only and should have little, if any, effect on the rest of your body. Diabetics may experience a slight temporary increase in blood sugar levels and should monitor their levels more carefully than usual for several days. Otherwise, we generally see very few side effects from injecting the carpal tunnel.

Most patients experience no problems or side effects following injection, and most also experience some relief from their symptoms. In short, injection is an effective and common form of initial treatment for carpal tunnel syndrome.

62 How will I know if the injection is working?

As with splinting (see Question 57), one of the first signs of improvement will be relief of your symptoms at night. In other words, you'll be able to sleep better because your hands will stop going numb and waking you up. This is a sign of improvement.

63 Is my doctor likely to recommend any other common nonsurgical treatments besides splinting and injection?

Other nonsurgical treatments that doctors who treat carpal tunnel syndrome may suggest include certain stretching exercises, anti-inflammatory drugs, and vitamins.

First, try doing the exercises described in the Appendix. These appear to be helpful in treating carpal tunnel syndrome as well as preventing it by reducing pressure in the carpal tunnel.

Second, you can try taking oral nonsteroidal anti-inflammatory drugs, often referred to as NSAIDs. These can give some improvement in the symptoms, especially if an inflammatory process such as rheumatoid arthritis is causing them. However, you should always follow package instructions regarding dosage and possible side effects.

Third, you can try taking 100 mg per day of vitamin B_6, which is often employed and appears to be useful in some cases. You can find it in any drugstore, either on its own or as part of a B-complex multivitamin. One month of vitamin B_6 should be enough to "top up your system." Be careful not to take more than this recommended dosage. More is not necessarily better.

Most doctors believe that avoiding flexed- or extended-wrist postures and reducing highly repetitive gripping activities can reduce the symptoms of carpal tunnel syndrome. This is a common form of treatment. If your work causes numbness in your hands, then changing your work might give you improvement. But, as I've mentioned before, changing jobs may be very disruptive to many people—in fact, you might find it easier to have surgery than to get a new job.

I often recommend that, for the first month or so of treatment, patients use the exercises and some of these medications in combination with night splinting and injection.

64 How long will my doctor recommend continuing to try nonsurgical treatments?

To some extent, this will depend on how much improvement you experienced and how much your symptoms continue to bother you.

For example, if splinting and injection give you dramatic relief for several months, it seems reasonable to repeat that same treatment at least one more time. But if you receive only a few weeks of benefit from those nonsurgical treatments, especially if you've repeated them with no further improvement, it probably won't be useful to continue with them for more than three months.

I usually recommend night splinting for at least a couple of months and will often try two injections spaced about six weeks apart before beginning to discuss surgery.

65 Can I try treating myself if I think I have carpal tunnel syndrome?

Please remember that this book is for educational and informational purposes only and can't take the place of a careful medical evaluation by your doctor.

If you're experiencing episodic hand numbness that also tends to wake you up at night, I see no harm in your wearing a night splint for a month. But if the splint doesn't relieve your symptoms, I urge you to see a doctor. Waiting while the symptoms grow worse will only make your condition harder and more complicated to treat.

66 Can I heal my carpal tunnel syndrome if I just rest my hands?

Like so many things in life, the answer is, "It depends."

Your doctor will usually recommend resting your hands and wrists in a splint if you're having symptoms of carpal tunnel syndrome. Also, reducing activities, especially those that provoke symptoms, can sometimes reduce your symptoms and in effect cure your carpal tunnel syndrome.

Some patients report that if they elevate their hands slightly by resting them on a pillow at night, they experience less numbness and fewer sleep disturbances. We assume that the slightly elevated position minimizes the accumulation of fluids, and thus pressure on the median nerve. However, if your carpal tunnel syndrome is due to swelling in the carpal tunnel or to a mass, resting your hands will not improve the symptoms.

67 I've read about laser treatments for carpal tunnel syndrome. Are they helpful?

Lasers can be used in two ways to treat carpal tunnel syndrome. The first is a treatment that aims a laser beam on the skin over the carpal tunnel, but I don't know why this could have any useful effect on the pressure on the median nerve.

Second, surgeons can use lasers as a high-technology scalpel. Because lasers can be aimed like a knife to cut fine lines through tissue, surgeons occasionally use them to cut the transverse carpal ligament in the endoscopic carpal tunnel surgery approach, discussed in depth in Part

Seven. Proponents of lasers say that they have an advantage because the laser cauterizes small blood vessels as it cuts. However, because the transverse carpal ligament has few blood vessels, bleeding is seldom a surgical issue.

68 *Why does pregnancy tend to aggravate carpal tunnel syndrome?*

Pregnant women often change their sleeping posture and also experience increases in fluid volume. Many note the onset of hand numbness at night during pregnancy and some notice it after delivery during breast-feeding. Symptoms can range from intermittent numbness at night to severe pain and numbness. In most cases, the symptoms disappear after delivery, so treatment is usually nonsurgical—night splinting or possibly an injection. Surgery is rarely needed unless the symptoms are severe and persist after delivery.

PART SIX

Surgical Solutions: Surgery for Carpal Tunnel Syndrome

✠

Introduction

Suppose that you've tried night splinting, injections, and even exercises and vitamin therapies, but your carpal tunnel syndrome fails to improve. At that point, your doctor will probably recommend surgery.

You won't be alone. According to one estimate, about 400,000 carpal tunnel releases are performed in the United States each year, making it the most common operation carried out by hand surgeons.

In my experience, most patients have one of two reactions to the idea of surgery. Some view the hand as a machine and see surgery as a process that will fix the hand and improve its functioning, rather like having a car repaired. These patients tend to be matter of fact about undergoing surgery and welcome any attempt to relieve their symptoms, even if the surgery involves some discomfort and inconvenience.

Other patients view their bodies as a deeply personal, intimate space and they consent to surgery only as a last distasteful attempt to heal their condition. For these patients to place their hands and their lives in the keeping of a surgeon and a surgical team requires the deepest level of trust. In my view, neither of these reactions is "right" or "wrong." Each of us is entitled to our own reactions. But because surgery is an incredibly personal experience, you should be sure to work with a surgeon who is aware of your feelings and can accept and work with you.

Once you're comfortable with the decision to have surgery, you may feel a sense of relief that you've finally made up your mind and are taking action to improve your condition. Try to remember that you'll be undergoing surgery only one time, but your surgeon and surgical team are experts and have operated on hundreds or thousands of patients.

Even if you aren't particularly bothered about the prospect of surgery, you may still worry about possible complications or things that might go wrong. Discuss any fears with your surgeon—and be sure that he or she is open to talking with you about those fears. For example, if you're a musician whose livelihood and identity depend on your hands, tell your surgeon about these issues. Similarly, if you've had previous surgeries that failed, you may have concerns about repeat surgeries that you wish to discuss.

You may find it reassuring to ask your surgeon about risks and about possible consequences such as scarring or nerve damage as a result of surgery. Having realistic information about the risks will allow you to weigh them against the high probability that your painful symptoms will improve.

The prospect of pain or discomfort during and after carpal tunnel surgery worries many patients. Again, you should express these concerns. These days, we have a more effective arsenal of pain medications than ever before. But you may find it comforting if I tell you that, when we ask for reports on pain after outpatient hand surgery, many patients report more pain before the surgery than after.

Try to do everything you can to make sure you're comfortable with your decision to have surgery. Avoid bottling up your anxieties. Discussing them with your surgeon as well as with your spouse, friends, and trusted others will relieve your mind and have a positive impact on your physical health as well as lessen any emotional stress. When you talk things through, you'll find that some of your concerns are genuine, while others are misconceptions.

It's normal and healthy to be upset about having surgery. A positive frame of mind is helpful. If you find yourself worrying excessively, review the problems that led you and your doctors to the decision and look forward to the relief from symptoms that you can expect to see after the surgery.

69 My family doctor says I need "carpal tunnel release." What does this involve?

As mentioned, *carpal tunnel release* is the usual term that refers to surgery done to release the pressure on the median nerve that causes the symptoms we know as carpal tunnel syndrome.

It involves making an incision in the skin and cutting the transverse carpal ligament, the strong band of tissue that forms the roof of the carpal tunnel. The ligament heals after the surgery but more loosely, creating about 25 percent more space in the carpal tunnel for the median nerve and other structures. The actual surgery is described in detail in Question 75.

70 When should I see a hand surgeon about my carpal tunnel syndrome?

Your family doctor or primary care physician is the obvious first person to see for any medical problem. However, if you've been working together on treatment but your symptoms haven't improved, your doctor may suggest referring you to a hand surgeon. If you're unhappy about your failure to improve, you may also ask for a referral.

If you don't have a regular family doctor and your insurance allows you to refer yourself to a specialist, you can consult with a hand surgeon about any hand problem. Hand surgeons are specialists who can evaluate your symptoms and provide the full range of treatments for carpal tunnel syndrome and other hand problems. Although hand surgeons perform surgery, they also have a great deal of experience with nonsurgical treatments.

71 How do hand surgeons receive their training?

Hand surgery is a subspecialty of surgery. To become a surgeon, medical school graduates enter a residency, or specialized training, in one of a number of areas such as general surgery, plastic surgery, or orthopedic surgery. Most residencies are four- or five-year programs.

When it comes to hand surgery, each of these "background specialties" may provide the student with some experience in hand surgery. Often, orthopedic and plastic surgery graduates gain enough training in hand surgery that they can safely perform many hand operations without further training. After completing any of these areas of background training, surgeons may choose to continue with their education and study hand surgery for another year. This extra year of intensive training is called a *fellowship*. After graduating from a fellowship program, surgeons typically think of themselves as hand surgeons and focus their interest in that area.

Hand surgeons may join one or more professional associations, such as the American Society for Surgery of the Hand or the American Association of Hand Surgeons. Surgeons who are not professional association members may be good at hand surgery, but those who do belong have demonstrated a special interest and training in the field. Whenever I'm asked to refer a patient to a surgeon outside my local area, I always choose surgeons who belong to one or both of these professional associations.

72 What's the best way to choose a surgeon for my carpal tunnel syndrome?

Traditionally, as mentioned, your family doctor will make an initial referral. If you don't have a regular doctor, there are several ways to find a good hand surgeon. You can ask family members and friends about experiences they may have had with hand surgery and hand surgeons. Your local medical association, or professional organizations such as the American Society for Surgery of the Hand or the American Association of Hand Surgeons, can give you a list of surgeons' names.

Many surgeons who are trained in general surgery, plastic surgery, or orthopedic surgery have an interest in hand surgery and may have experience with carpal tunnel surgery. But if I needed surgery for carpal tunnel syndrome, I would choose a hand surgeon to do the operation.

I should add that you, as a patient, won't really be able to judge by your conversations with your surgeon the quality of the surgery he will perform or the level of his knowledge. However, most hand surgeons are skilled at hand surgery and passionate about the hand.

What you *can* observe is the surgeon's behavior, and how she deals with and treats you and other people in the office. If you have reservations about any surgeon with whom you consult—if you don't like her "bedside manner," look for another doctor. You're going to be going through a lot, and you need to feel that you and your surgeon are on the same "team" and that you're both comfortable.

Make sure the surgeon you choose takes time to listen to you and to answer all your questions. If a surgeon is too busy to explain things, is rude to you, or seems to minimize your concerns and not take them seriously, look for someone else. There is a surplus of surgeons of all kinds, so you have your choice.

73 *What should I do if the idea of having surgery scares me?*

First of all, you should feel normal. The prospect of having surgery— of having someone cut into your hand with a knife—frightens most people. Keep in mind, however, that you're deciding to have surgery because you have a problem that bothers you every day, and perhaps every night, of your life. You're having trouble sleeping, you can't have fun with activities you like, clumsiness in your hands is interfering with your work, and you've tried all the nonsurgical treatments available with no improvement.

If you know your surgeon through your office visits and you feel satisfied and confident about his or her ability, you should be able to place your trust in your surgeon. Keep in mind that carpal tunnel release is one of the most common surgical procedures performed these days and that your surgeon has done it hundreds of times. Patients rarely experience problems after carpal tunnel release, and you're likely to be in the vast majority who sail through the operation and postoperative care—and who experience total relief from symptoms.

74 Is there more than one type of operation for carpal tunnel release?

Surgeons today use two major forms of carpal tunnel release: the traditional surgical treatment, also known as the open technique, which is sometimes now performed with a smaller incision than was customary (small-incision technique); and endoscopic carpal tunnel release.

In the open technique, the surgeon makes an incision on the inside surface of the wrist and cuts the transverse carpal ligament. This technique first came into use in the 1940s and has been employed successfully ever since. Over time it has undergone some modifications, but it continues to be the most common surgical technique for carpal tunnel release.

The endoscopic technique has become more common in the past ten years with the development of the endoscope, a family of tiny fiber-optic scopes that allow doctors and surgeons to view many parts of the body that could never before be seen without invasive surgery.

In endoscopic carpal tunnel release, the surgeon makes one or more small incisions into the wrist above the carpal tunnel and, looking through the endoscope, cuts the transverse carpal ligament with a tiny, specially designed scalpel. As the endoscopic approach has come into wider use, surgeons have developed variations in the technique, such as carrying out the surgery through a small incision in the palm or at the wrist crease, or sometimes in both locations.

Over time, even some surgeons who preferred to continue using the traditional approach realized the advantages of using smaller surgical incisions. Because smaller incisions can lessen postsurgery discomfort from cut nerves in the incision area and can speed recovery time, surgeons began using smaller incisions even in the open technique. They now use the terms *small-incision technique* or *mini-incision technique* to describe this approach, as depicted in Figure 10.

Figure 10 shows the changes in incision length and location over the past twenty years. The incision for an endoscopic surgery is usually even shorter than the smallest incision shown here. In addition, locating the incision closer to the ulnar (outer) side of the wrist places it in

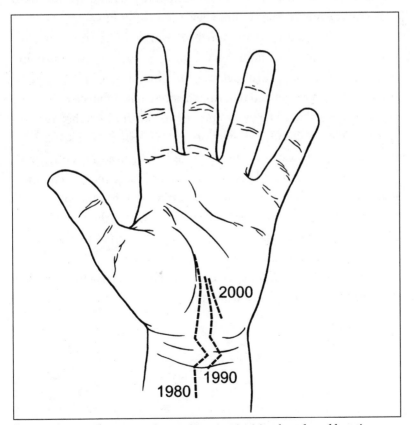

Figure 10. Changes in carpal tunnel surgery incision length and location

a location where fewer of the small branches of the median and ulnar nerves are likely to be cut. Because it's impossible to avoid cutting small nerve branches in the area, most patients experience some post-surgery sensitivity around the incision and scar. The smaller incisions involved in endoscopic releases seem to result in less sensitivity.

Variations exist within both major types of surgery. For example, I work with one surgeon who uses an open surgical technique that avoids cutting the transverse carpal ligament. Instead, he makes a small incision at the wrist on the forearm side and removes the synovial tissue that lines the flexor tendons (described in detail in Part Two) as they enter the carpal tunnel. This procedure, called a *synovectomy,* reduces the volume of tissue in the carpal tunnel and creates more room for the median nerve, thus alleviating symptoms.

In addition to these common procedures, some surgeons have worked with experimental surgery techniques such as inserting a tiny balloon into the carpal tunnel and then inflating it in the hope of stretching the ligament and relieving the pressure on the median nerve.

All surgeons have one or two procedures with which they're most comfortable. I recommend that you and your surgeon discuss what type of surgical procedure is planned, and that you also educate yourself about the positive and possible negative consequences of choosing that procedure. All three major techniques—traditional open, small incision, and endoscopic—are widely performed in the United States at this time. Most surgeons will use the open or small-incision technique; some will also use the endoscopic technique.

The pros and cons of the endoscopic and traditional approaches are discussed in more detail in Part Seven.

75 Can you give me a step-by-step description of what will actually happen during carpal tunnel surgery? How long does the operation usually take?

First, a member of the medical team will anesthetize your hand and arm and wash your hand with a disinfectant soap. A high-tech blood pressure cuff called a tourniquet will be placed around your arm or forearm to stop blood circulation to the hand, and your arm will be covered with towels and sheets called *drapes*. These serve to isolate the area where the surgery will take place.

Your surgeon may draw a line on the skin where the incision is planned. He or she will then hold your hand up in the air and may wrap an elastic bandage around your hand and forearm from the fingertips to the tourniquet. The pressure from the bandage milks the blood out of your arm, which minimizes bleeding and makes it easier for the surgeon to see the physical structures in the wrist during the surgery. Some surgeons don't wrap the arm but just lift it to let the blood drain down by gravity.

After inflating the tourniquet cuff, the surgeon makes the incision in the location chosen and gently spreads open the fatty tissue under the skin until the transverse carpal ligament, the roof of the carpal tunnel, becomes visible. The surgeon then cuts the ligament, which is the essence of the surgery. After the carpal tunnel roof is cut, there's no more pressure on the median nerve, and the healing process can begin.

After cutting the ligament, the surgeon will check the median nerve and the degree of compression, and will also feel around the carpal tunnel to see if there is any swelling or mass pressing on the nerve. The motor branch, which is the area at the beginning of the palm where the median nerve branches, is checked because sometimes it passes in a small tunnel of its own and must also be released. Any thickened synovial tissue around the flexor tendons may also be removed.

Finally, the tourniquet is deflated and the surgical site compressed with absorbent pieces of gauze, called *sponges*, to control any bleeding. The surgeon will use an electrical device called a *cautery* that uses heat to seal or cauterize the ends of any small blood vessels that might be bleeding before closing the incision with stitches and covering the site with a light dressing or bandage.

The details of this general procedure may vary slightly depending on the particular anesthetic and surgical technique the surgeon prefers.

The endoscopic procedure, described in the previous question, is similar until the incision is made, at which point the surgeon uses the endoscope to carry out the rest of the operation.

In North America, carpal tunnel release is almost always performed on an outpatient basis, which means that you come in, undergo the surgery, and go home the same day. The actual operation, whether using the traditional or the endoscopic approach, usually takes about thirty minutes, but with paperwork, anesthesia time, and recovery time, you should count on about half a day.

76 How many stitches will I need? When will my doctor take them out?

The number of stitches, or sutures, needed to close the incision will depend on its length. The endoscopic and small-incision techniques may require as few as three or four sutures, while the traditional open-style incision may require as many as fifteen or twenty.

Surgeons usually expect to leave the sutures in place for about two weeks, depending on individual patients' variations in healing time. Most sutures used today are made of a monofilament synthetic material that is nonabsorbing and nonreactive, meaning that they don't dissolve and they don't cause inflammatory reactions. Because adults are seldom apprehensive about having stitches removed, hand surgeons use these sutures rather than the dissolving ones for carpal tunnel surgery in adults. When it comes to children, however, surgeons may use quick-dissolving sutures because children can become upset about the idea of having stitches removed. Dissolving sutures sometimes cause a slightly greater skin reaction, but they're less stressful for the child.

To remove the stitches, the doctor or nurse first wipes them with an alcohol pad, then lifts up one side of the stitch with a small pair of tweezers called forceps and cuts the stitch with a pair of scissors. The stitch is then pulled out.

If for some reason your stitches must be removed before the incision has healed, your doctor can use tape to keep the edges together. After about three weeks, most carpal tunnel incisions have healed enough to withstand the stresses and forces placed on your hand by day-to-day activities.

Never try removing stitches yourself. If you use nonsterile instruments, you could cause a serious hand infection.

77 Will my surgeon give me pain medications after carpal tunnel surgery?

If you're like most patients, you'll experience little severe pain after carpal tunnel surgery. Because this is an outpatient procedure, your doctor will prescribe oral medication, which can range in strength from over-the-counter analgesics to powerful narcotics. Your doctor will choose the most appropriate medication for you.

The most common nonprescription medications include common aspirin (acetylsalicylic acid or ASA), acetaminophen (Tylenol and related brand names), and nonsteroidal anti-inflammatory drugs (NSAIDs) such as ibuprofen (Advil and related brand names).

Aspirin works well for many types of pain, but it's not considered strong enough to be used after most operations, so it's unlikely that your surgeon will suggest aspirin alone after carpal tunnel surgery. The same is true of the weaker nonprescription dosages of acetaminophen and ibuprofen sold over the counter.

The main side effect experienced by patients who take aspirin or NSAIDs is stomach irritation. I always advise patients to take these medications with food and caution them not to take them if they have any history of ulcers or gastrointestinal bleeding, aspirin-induced asthma, or, of course, any prior allergic reactions.

Your surgeon is more likely to prescribe one of several stronger narcotic pain medications after carpal tunnel surgery. These drugs, most of which are derived from opium, act on special chemical receptors in the brain to reduce pain. They're called narcotics because they tend to make people drowsy.

The most commonly prescribed pain medications for carpal tunnel surgery are Tylenol with codeine, hydrocodone, or oxycodone. These are powerful narcotic "cousins" that are chemically similar to morphine and do a good job of controlling pain after outpatient surgery. Oxycodone is the strongest of the three but also has the highest potential for addiction and abuse. For this reason, your surgeon is likely to prescribe either hydrocodone, commonly known as Vicodan or Lortab, or Tylenol with codeine (Tylenol 3).

The two most common pain medications administered to hospital patients after surgery are morphine and Demerol, both very effective analgesics. However, they're usually injected into the muscles rather than given in pill form. If used at all following carpal tunnel surgery, they would be administered on a very short-term basis in the recovery room if for some reason a patient were experiencing unusual postoperative pain.

78 Will I have to wear a splint after carpal tunnel surgery?

Surgeons differ on the benefits of wearing a splint after surgery.

In the past, many surgeons kept the patient's wrist splinted for about two weeks after surgery and took the splint off when the stitches were removed. Some surgeons believe that a splint will keep the wrist from flexing, which in turn prevents the flexor tendons pushing forward against the nerve. Other surgeons see no need for splinting and believe in allowing the patient to move the hand and fingers freely after surgery. This is particularly true when the endoscopic or small-incision technique has been used.

I don't think that splinting during the day is necessary after carpal tunnel surgery. I use a soft dressing only and ask patients to wear a loose splint at night to keep their wrists in a relatively straight position; but obviously, you should follow your surgeon's advice.

79 How long will it take for the incision to heal?

Most incisions made for carpal tunnel surgery will heal within two weeks after the operation. During this time, if the stitches come out, the incision can easily split open. After the first two weeks, healing should be well underway, and by four weeks after surgery, I allow and even encourage patients to perform all activities with their hands.

Occasionally, the scar can become red and thickened. We call this a *hypertrophic scar,* and it can take six months to a year to flatten and become soft. Most scars blend into the creases of the hand, sometimes so well that we have trouble even locating them in the future.

80 Which anesthetics work best for carpal tunnel surgery, and what are their advantages and disadvantages?

Surgeons commonly use one of four types of anesthesia to prevent pain or discomfort during carpal tunnel surgery: local anesthesia; one of two forms of regional anesthesia, intravenous anesthesia or brachial plexus block anesthesia; or general anesthesia. Each has advantages and disadvantages.

Local anesthesia is the simplest and easiest to administer. If you've ever had dental work or a cut sutured, you've probably received a local anesthetic. Either the surgeon or the team member responsible for anesthesia, who might be an M.D. anesthesiologist but will more likely be a nurse anesthetist, uses a small needle to inject the anesthetic into the carpal tunnel area in much the same way that your doctor might have anesthetized the area before injecting cortisone in the initial stages of treating your carpal tunnel syndrome (see Part Five). Because local anesthetics block the transmission of nerve impulses in the area, they offer good pain relief. Sometimes local anesthetic medication is combined with adrenaline to constrict the small blood vessels and reduce any bleeding. Your surgeon may also add some sedating medication intravenously to make you feel more comfortable.

Local anesthetics are quite safe and, if not used with sedation, leave patients awake and alert immediately after the surgery. Another advantage is that local anesthetics usually don't require an anesthetist, which lowers the cost of the operation. Their disadvantages include some pain during the injection itself and possibly some discomfort from the pressure of the tourniquet, although carpal tunnel surgery is usually completed in such a short time that this is not too painful. Some surgeons also feel that, because the anesthetic is a fluid, it can cause some swelling and distortion of the tissue in the area. The benefits of local anesthetics compared to their risks make them a common choice for carpal tunnel surgery.

Both the second and third methods mentioned previously involve regional anesthesia. In intravenous regional anesthesia, the anesthesiologist will start one intravenous drip in a vein of the arm that will have surgery to deliver the anesthetic medication and a second one in the other arm to deliver medication for sedation.

A double tourniquet keeps the anesthetic in the arm, where it diffuses into the tissues from the local veins and completely anesthetizes the area. In addition to the anesthesia, I sometimes add a sedating drug if the patient prefers it or if the anesthetist thinks it desirable. When the tourniquet is removed after the surgery, the anesthetic effect wears off quickly and the hand and arm regain their feeling and motion in minutes.

Intravenous anesthesia is safe and efficient, but, like all procedures, it carries some risk. For one thing, a relatively large amount of local anesthesia must be injected into the veins to numb the entire hand and arm. If this much local anesthetic were injected directly into the bloodstream without a tourniquet, it might cause side effects such as a seizure or an adverse effect on the heart. Hence, the double tourniquet is very important because it provides double safety for the technique. Both tourniquets are tested and inflated before any medication is injected.

In the brachial plexus block, the other type of regional anesthesia, a local anesthetic is injected into the cluster of nerves under the collarbone and armpit area that provide sensation and muscle power to the arm and hand. This injection blocks the nerves and makes the entire arm numb. It shares some of the advantages of the intravenous block in that the patient remains conscious throughout the surgery and thus feels better soon afterward. The anesthetist can also add a sedating drug to allay the patient's anxiety about the injections and the operation. One disadvantage of the brachial plexus block is that it can irritate the nerves and cause tingling and electrical shocks in the hand, arm, or armpit that may persist after the surgery and occasionally require physical therapy.

The possibility, slight and temporary though it might be, of causing symptoms that resemble the condition the surgery is trying to relieve is enough to dissuade many surgeons from using the brachial plexus block for carpal tunnel surgery.

In general anesthesia, patients are "put to sleep" temporarily to prevent pain and movement during surgery. An anesthetist inserts a needle into the vein of your arm and injects medication that makes you unconscious and unaware of anything going on around you. General anesthesia slows your breathing, so the anesthetist will usually pass a tube down your windpipe to help you breathe and protect your airway.

General anesthesia is very safe, but it's slightly riskier than the other types. Sometimes patients feel nauseated after coming out of general anesthesia, and it can take several hours for the anesthetic to completely work its way out of your system. Newer drugs are associated with much less nausea but still require longer recovery times than does local anesthesia. General anesthesia is not commonly used for carpal tunnel surgery, but it is a reasonable choice for patients who prefer not to be aware of the procedure.

81 If I have carpal tunnel syndrome in both wrists, can I have both hands operated on at the same time?

We usually recommend surgery on only one hand at a time for several reasons. First, we've observed that sometimes after a patient has surgery on one hand, the other hand improves without surgery. We're not sure why this should be so, but it does happen. One obvious explanation may be that, when the hand that has been operated on improves, the patient can use it more and this gives the other hand a chance to rest and perhaps heal on its own. Some surgeons also believe that the nerves of the body are interconnected in such a way that relieving one area of compression may improve the health of other related nerves.

Second, as in any surgery, unusual but serious complications can arise after hand surgery. Because we can't know in advance whether you might be susceptible to a complication, it's wise to expose only one hand at a time to that risk.

Third, because surgery is a big step, it's probably wise to undergo surgery in one hand before having both hands treated.

There's one other obvious reason: If you have surgery on both hands, you'll find it almost impossible to care for yourself in the immediate postoperative period.

Still, I'm not totally opposed to operating on both hands at the same time and will discuss this with patients in advance if that's what they want.

82 How long will it take for my symptoms to improve after carpal tunnel surgery?

Most patients notice some improvement almost immediately, barring any pain or limitations due to the surgery itself. You may notice an improvement in the numbness that very night, and patients often comment that they find themselves sleeping better right away. The aftereffects of the surgery usually wane within the first two weeks after the procedure. Because I always use the smallest possible incision for the surgery and have patients wear a splint only at night, in most cases they can begin using their hands for light activities the day after the operation. A few days later, I ask patients to take off the large dressing and protect the stitches with a couple of ordinary bandages. Two weeks after the surgery, patients come to the office and have the stitches removed. At this time, they can use their hands for all light activities.

In my experience, by the time of their two-week follow-up visit, many patients are no longer experiencing any of their preoperative symptoms, and the rest of their recovery consists of gradually resuming using their hands. Within a month after surgery, many patients are carrying out most of their regular activities with total comfort. After three months, most patients are completely recovered and report no numbness or tingling.

83 Will I need physical therapy or rehabilitation after carpal tunnel surgery?

Few patients require physical therapy after carpal tunnel release. However, if you do experience symptoms after surgery, therapy can be of great benefit. It can increase the motion in your wrist and fingers, make the scar less sensitive, improve your ability to use your hand in day-to-day activities, and make returning to work easier and more comfortable.

PART SEVEN

Tradition and Innovation: The Benefits and Risks of Traditional and Endoscopic Surgery

Introduction

Although I discussed endoscopic and traditional open carpal tunnel surgery in Part Six, it's important to examine this issue in more depth here because the endoscopic approach is not only a surgical technique but also a new surgical philosophy.

Endoscopic, or minimally invasive, surgery uses small incisions to perform operations that previously required longer incisions and were thus more invasive and traumatic to the body. The advantage of endoscopic surgery is that patients appear to experience less trauma and, it is hoped, a faster recovery time. Minimally invasive surgery is now widely accepted and is being used for all types of procedures, from cardiac bypass surgery to face-lifts, but at times it has been an uphill struggle.

In the early 1980s, orthopedic surgeons began using fiber-optic scopes called *arthroscopes* to look into the knee joint and to diagnose and treat injuries and diseases in that area. Inserting the arthroscope required only a small incision, and arthroscopic surgery became a popular technique for use on athletes because it allowed an earlier return to sports and other activities. At about the same time, gynecologists began using endoscopic surgery to study women's ovaries and reproductive organs and to tie off the fallopian tubes to prevent pregnancy.

The general surgical community resisted the endoscopic approach, though, especially for abdominal surgery, for quite a while. "Wounds heal from side to side, not end to end" and "There's no such thing as a small incision, only a small surgeon" sum up the orthodox surgical view of minimally invasive surgery at that time.

Gradually, however, orthopedic surgeons began using arthroscopes to work on other joints, such as the wrist. The technology advanced further as smaller and smaller scopes and instruments were developed. Endoscopic surgery came into the public eye when cholecystectomy, or gallbladder removal, became the first general surgical procedure to be commonly performed using endoscopic techniques.

Although the surgical community resisted it, over time it became clear that this approach was safe and that it not only resulted in faster recovery times but also produced smaller scars than "open" removal of the gallbladder. After intense media interest, the endoscopic technique finally won out both in the operating room and in the public eye. This primed the public for other forms of endoscopic surgery, so orthopedic surgeons skilled in the endoscopic technique from arthroscopy of small joints, including the wrist, began applying it to carpal tunnel surgery.

Still, endoscopic carpal tunnel surgery has a history of controversy. The surgical community had doubts about the design of the earliest instruments, which were withdrawn from the market and reengineered. Because the anatomy of the hand is so dense and so vital, many surgeons were also concerned about the risk of injury to nerves, arteries, and tendons.

Soon after the commencement of endoscopic surgery, variations of the instrumentation and procedures were introduced. Within a few years of its introduction in the early 1980s, roughly a quarter of the hand surgeons in the United States were performing it.

Has endoscopic carpal tunnel surgery turned out to be better than the traditional "open" technique? At first, practitioners hoped that it would let patients return to work and other activities sooner, but early research failed to prove this point. The procedure has endured, however, as surgeons discovered that it was not dramatically riskier than the traditional approach.

In addition, as mentioned, one effect of the endoscopic technique has been a change in thinking about incisions, with many surgeons using smaller incisions than in the past because smaller incisions appear to decrease the risk of injury to the small nerves in the skin, and thus result in less scar sensitivity.

At this point, do we know whether the endoscopic approach offers any benefits over the standard technique? I believe that the final answer isn't yet in, nor am I sure about the ultimate place of endoscopy in hand surgery. I do feel that it's a reasonable technique when performed by an experienced hand surgeon. Surgeons who perform it regularly have become very good at it, and I believe that the risks of the procedure are balanced by its potential benefits for patients who want or need to get back to activities as soon as possible.

84 What are endoscopes, and how do surgeons use them in carpal tunnel surgery?

An endoscope is a fiber-optic scope that can be placed inside a body cavity. Endoscopic carpal tunnel surgery uses a fiber-optic instrument especially designed to be used in the wrist area to release the carpal tunnel.

The surgeon uses the endoscope to see the surgical area through a small incision. In reality, the fiber-optics of the endoscope are connected to a camera, and the surgery is performed while watching the surgical field on a TV monitor. To take advantage of this, instruments have been developed that can be used through the endoscope or through small adjacent incisions.

85 What are the advantages and risks of endoscopic carpal tunnel surgery compared to the traditional and small-incision approaches?

As mentioned in the introduction to this section, these issues are still being debated and researched. The main advantage of the endoscopic approach is that the procedure can be carried out using a smaller incision, which may hurt less and allow for faster healing and an earlier return to activity afterward. Endoscopic surgery not only involves a smaller incision than does the traditional open approach; the incision is made in an area where there's not much contact when patients use the hand to grip objects.

Also, as mentioned, when the skin of the hand is cut due to a laceration or a surgical incision, tiny nerves in the skin are also cut. While these nerves are healing, they sometimes become tender, especially if they're in the immediate area of the scar. This is seldom more than a minor inconvenience, and most patients manage with some massage until time passes and sensitivity improves. Occasionally, however, the cut nerves can produce a very tender scar, and the tenderness slows recovery and the ability to use the hand vigorously.

In addition, because the surgery takes place under the skin, some of the fatty padding just under the skin remains in place, and this may make the surgical site more comfortable. However, the tiny size of the incision and the use of the endoscope do not give as good a view of the carpal tunnel area as does the longer incision used in the traditional open technique. Because the surgeon sees the surgical area only through the fiber-optic scope, the view is not complete. In fact, some endoscopic techniques don't allow a view of the median nerve at all, and this is of concern to surgeons because they feel it increases the risk of cutting the median nerve or other important structures. The endoscopic approach may thus involve a somewhat greater risk of damage to the nerves, tendons, and arteries in the hand, though surgeons who are experts in the technique dispute this point, and the research is not definitive.

Either technique, endoscopic or open, creates some risk of cutting the median nerve, causing a degree of permanent numbness in the hand. It may be that the relatively less complete visibility offered by the endoscopic approach increases this risk. There's also some concern about whether incomplete release, in which the transverse carpal ligament is not completely cut, may occur more often with the endoscopic technique. The limited research carried out so far hasn't resolved these questions.

In sum, both techniques, when performed by experienced hand surgeons, are safe and give excellent relief from carpal tunnel syndrome in most patients.

86 Will traditional, endoscopic, and small-incision carpal tunnel surgery all give me the same results?

We still don't know whether one technique is clearly superior to the other two. As noted, the perceived benefits of the smaller incision used in endoscopic surgery have encouraged some surgeons to use smaller incisions in the open, nonendoscopic technique as well. Surgeons feel that the smaller incision offers some of the benefits of the endoscopic approach without the possible risk of cutting the median nerve or other problems. Still, the traditional open technique has a long and positive track record despite the disadvantages of a longer scar that may result in more scar tenderness and a slight delay in return to activity.

In the small-incision technique, the incision is usually placed in the palm of the hand. Because the surgeon can actually see the important structures of the palm, such as the median nerve branches and the large blood vessels, they can be kept out of the way as the surgery proceeds. The surgeon locates the edge of the transverse carpal ligament and then cuts it, working under the skin from the palm toward the wrist. Specialized instruments have been developed to make this technique easier.

So we now have three options: traditional open technique, open small-incision technique, and endoscopic technique.

PART EIGHT

Complications and Problems: When Carpal Tunnel Release Fails

Introduction

Suppose that you've gone ahead with carpal tunnel surgery, but you're still having symptoms or have experienced complications. What should you do now?

Your first instinct might well be to blame your surgeon. You may feel that she must have done something wrong if the surgery didn't work. Your second thought may be to blame yourself for having made a bad decision. You may even start feeling that you never should have agreed to the operation.

Before you go too far down these roads, stop for a moment. First of all, your surgeon does want you to get better. In spite of all the complexity of the medical marketplace, the insurance industry, managed care, and organized medicine, all doctors want their patients to get better.

Before the surgery, you got to know your doctor and had confidence in his ability to help you. You realized that although surgery is never a sure thing as far as guaranteeing a complete recovery, your doctor recommended it for you because of your unique situation and the likelihood that it could help your symptoms. You thought through your options and considered each of them. Even if the surgery did not work, *you made the correct decision.* Hindsight is always 20/20.

So blaming yourself is a waste of energy. Suppose you were facing the same choice again, without the benefits of hindsight. Going ahead with the surgery would *still* be the best decision. None of us can predict the future; if we could, we'd all be making fortunes in the stock market.

Should you dump your surgeon and try someone new? Should you get a lawyer? These are certainly gut-wrenching questions, but I suggest that you stop dwelling on the past, accept that you made the right decision in having surgery, and develop a positive plan for healing your hand and moving on with your life.

Once again, the first step in solving your problem is for your doctor to consider your medical history and perform a physical examination. Your doctor will need to evaluate whether you had carpal tunnel syndrome and the surgery failed to give you improvement, or whether you did not have carpal tunnel syndrome after all, but some other condition. Your doctor may suggest getting a second opinion, and you should feel free to ask for one. I strongly recommend second opinions before patients undergo another carpal tunnel release.

The surgeon who operated on you is still in the best position to help you. Your surgeon is familiar with your case, knows how you respond, has examined you and your hand on several occasions, and was able to observe the median nerve directly during your first operation. If you have any concerns about the advice your surgeon gives you, or if the advice indicates that you would have to live with significant symptoms or make difficult choices about your future, such as leaving your occupation, you should definitely get a second opinion.

At the very least, take time to think about these decisions for as long as it takes to feel comfortable, and talk with your family, your friends, your boss, your minister, priest, or rabbi, and anyone else whose opinion you value. Take all the time you need to be satisfied that you're making the best decision for your own future.

Suffering from surgical complications is stressful, not just for you but also for your surgeon and for the relationship between the two of you. However, the best way to resolve difficulties after surgery is to develop a plan with your doctor. What you've already been through together will help get you through those problems. You must weigh the advantages of that ongoing relationship against the possible pluses and minuses of seeking out a new surgeon who might be a stranger to your case.

If difficulties arise, try to approach them in a thoughtful, careful manner. Learn about the problem, ask questions of your surgeon, and remember that you're both on the same side. You both want your hands to be comfortable and to work well.

87 How often does carpal tunnel surgery give complete relief from symptoms?

The chances for a complete recovery after carpal tunnel surgery are very good, with about 90 percent of patients experiencing complete, long-lasting relief of their symptoms. Exact statistics are hard to obtain because carpal tunnel surgery is so common and is often done on an outpatient basis.

If your symptoms don't improve after surgery, however, you should go back to your hand surgeon without delay. Your doctor will again take your medical history and perform a physical examination because assessing your symptoms before and after the operation are important in determining the cause of your ongoing problems. It's likely that the doctor will want to repeat your nerve tests, or perform these tests if they weren't done earlier. Repeating the electrical tests may reveal that there has not been a complete return to normal even in patients who are symptom free, but if the nerve tests show increased changes, this would be cause for concern.

In short, your surgeon will try to determine the cause of your ongoing symptoms and what further treatment might help you.

88 What does it mean if my symptoms don't get better after surgery, or if they improve for a while and then get worse?

There are several causes of continued symptoms after carpal tunnel surgery. It was once thought that the most common cause of continuing symptoms was the surgeon's failure to completely release the carpal tunnel. This is a potential concern in the endoscopic and small-incision approaches because the surgeon does not have as long an incision to look through as in the traditional technique. However, research has shown that patients' symptoms can improve even if only the deep fibers of the transverse carpal ligament are released, so I don't believe that incomplete release accounts for the persistence of symptoms.

In my view, the most likely reason for failure to get complete relief from carpal tunnel surgery is that other causes are responsible for a patient's symptoms. When the carpal tunnel is released, any symptoms coming from the carpal tunnel will resolve, but other sources of symptoms have not been affected and will leave the patient with continued problems. The symptoms could be from another area of nerve compression or from some other source of pain, such as arthritis.

In spite of your doctor's best effort to ensure that the cause of your symptoms is the carpal tunnel, there will always be some uncertainty. One explanation, as mentioned, may be that the nerve is compressed at another location. The nerve is "hard-wired" to your brain, so if it's compressed anywhere along its length, your brain will perceive the location of the compression to be the hand and will feel the numbness there. So if you have nerve compression from arthritis of the spine or some other cause, release of the nerve at the carpal tunnel will not eliminate your symptoms.

Patients with severe carpal tunnel syndrome may have nerve compression that is too advanced to allow the nerve to recover even after it is released. For example, there may be scarring within the nerve itself from the effects of long-lasting, severe compression. However, I believe this condition is rare and that carpal tunnel release can give good relief of symptoms even in severe carpal tunnel syndrome.

Finally, it's possible that new symptoms that arise after surgery could be the result of the surgery itself; for example, if the small nerves in the skin are damaged. Injury to the median nerve or to its large branches has been reported after both open and endoscopic carpal tunnel release. Needless to say, surgeons take every precaution to avoid this, but some rare anatomic variations exist that can increase the risk of nerve injury during surgery (see Questions 91 and 92).

Some patients experience temporary relief of symptoms after surgery followed by a recurrence of problems. After carpal tunnel release, the transverse carpal ligament heals with about 25 percent more space in the carpal tunnel. If you feel relief of your numbness after surgery, this suggests that you probably did have carpal tunnel syndrome and that the surgery relieved the nerve compression. The return of symptoms after a period of relief—recurrent carpal tunnel syndrome—could be from some underlying condition such as rheumatoid arthritis or from a return to vigorous activity, but the cause is usually unknown. If you develop recurrent carpal tunnel syndrome, your hand surgeon will reevaluate you and may recommend some or all of the nonsurgical treatments discussed in Question 93.

89 What complications are associated with carpal tunnel surgery?

Complications are undesirable results that sometimes occur after surgical procedures despite surgeons' best efforts to avoid them.

We usually group complications into those related to anesthesia, those related to any type of surgery, and those related to the specific operation you undergo. Complications can happen in any of these areas; luckily, they are rare. Still, barring emergency operations, you're wise to be aware of and to understand the possible complications of any operation before you decide to have it. That way you can consider the operation and its possible ramifications and make the best decision for yourself.

When surgeons discuss the possible complications of an operation, they want to give you enough information to help you make a wise decision without scaring you or causing information overload. If you tell your surgeon that you want every detail, she will start by saying, "You could die." This is true. Death is unlikely, but it can happen during any operation, just as it is a possibility in many everyday activities such as driving, riding a bicycle, and even eating. Most surgeons will focus on telling you about the rare complications that can be serious, and about the mild complications that are common.

I believe that all patients should be aware that surgery is never a "sure thing" for the complete relief of symptoms. Even with the most thorough evaluation, surgeons can never be positive that surgery will give complete relief. However, you might take comfort in the fact that your surgeon will have factored the probability of success into the "equation" before recommending surgery.

In general, carpal tunnel surgery is very safe and complications are rare. When brachial plexus block anesthesia is used in carpal tunnel surgery, I tell patients that they may experience some sensitivity around the brachial plexus after the operation. All patients are told that there's a slight chance of infection after surgery and that they may feel some sensitivity in the scar.

Some of the possible complications specific to carpal tunnel release include swelling, infection of the hand, severe pain, and scar sensitivity. Some degree of swelling is likely to occur following any surgery involving the hand. On occasion, this swelling is enough to cause stiffness and to limit wrist and/or finger motion. If this occurs, your surgeon will encourage you to move your fingers and may suggest physiotherapy (rehabilitation, also known as physical therapy).

Infection is a possibility after any type of surgery. The risk for serious infection after carpal tunnel surgery is very low, less than one in one thousand. The signs of infection include redness and firmness of the wound, unusual pain, swelling and stiffness of the hand and fingers, and drainage of pus from the surgery site. Infection after carpal tunnel surgery is usually mild and superficial and can be treated with oral antibiotics. On rare occasions when an infection is more serious, the surgeon will remove the sutures and open the wound to allow the infection to drain. Sometimes surgeons recommend that this be done in the operating room under anesthesia so that the surgical site can be washed thoroughly and cleaned with surgical gauze. After the cleaning, the surgeon usually leaves the incision open and allows it to heal without stitches.

Pain soon after surgery can be considered a complication because it's undesirable and can usually be prevented. In addition, it is an important symptom that can tell you and your doctor that something isn't quite right and needs to be checked. But as mentioned, patients seldom complain of severe pain after carpal tunnel surgery.

Experiencing some pain and sensitivity around the incision is common in the weeks after surgery. A condition called "pillar pain," which involves pain and tenderness at the sides of the carpal tunnel in the area of the scaphoid bone on one side and the hamate bone on the other side, can be treated with ultrasound by a physical therapist.

Prolonged pain after carpal tunnel surgery is rare, but because the operation releases the median nerve and pain is one of the sensations transmitted by nerves, prolonged pain can occur after surgery. If you're still having pain several months after the procedure, you should ask your surgeon for a careful evaluation. Your doctor will try to determine if your pain is due to another cause, such as a pinched nerve in the neck or another location. There may even be repeat nerve compression at the site of the surgery.

As mentioned several times, the endoscopic and small-incision techniques for carpal tunnel surgery are thought to result in less scar sensitivity. If you experience sensitivity in the area of the healing incision, self-massage or treatment by a physical therapist usually takes care of the problem.

90 My surgeon mentioned reflex sympathetic dystrophy as a possible complication of carpal tunnel surgery. What is this, and how is it treated?

Reflex sympathetic dystrophy, or RSD, is a rare but unpredictable complication of the sympathetic nervous system characterized by hand pain, stiffness, and swelling, which causes patients to have difficulty regaining use of their hands. It can occur after any type of hand injury or surgery, including carpal tunnel release, but no one really knows what causes it.

We treat RSD by first ruling out any other possible conditions of the hand. We then eliminate any other ongoing sources of pain that can be corrected. Following this, we use physical therapy in the form of gentle mobilization and use of the hand. We also focus on maintaining range of motion of the joints of the hand, shoulder, and elbow. The third aspect of treatment requires the help of the anesthetist. Because RSD involves the sympathetic nervous system, one commonly used treatment blocks those nerves with a local anesthetic at a place where they are accessible in the neck. If these local anesthetic blocks are effective, a series of daily blocks can be carried out.

After attempting one or two sympathetic blocks, your doctor will be able to tell if they're helping and may recommend a series of six or eight if they are working well. If you experience no improvement after one or two blocks, this treatment is unlikely to be of great benefit. RSD can resolve itself over time, but often persists with permanent stiffness and pain.

91 Is it possible to injure a nerve during carpal tunnel surgery?

Although surgeons of course try to avoid nerve injuries during surgery, they are a well-documented complication of carpal tunnel release. The median nerve is the largest nerve encountered during the surgery. As was discussed in Part Seven, surgeons can clearly see the median nerve in the traditional open surgical approach, but it isn't as visible when using the endoscopic and small-incision techniques. This is seldom a problem, but given the possibility of individual anatomical variations, your median nerve could lie in an unexpected position that would make it susceptible to injury.

Other nerves in the hand can also be injured. The palmar sensory branch of the median nerve, a sensory nerve to the skin of the palm, branches from the median nerve about 8 cm above the wrist crease. This nerve lies under the skin in the region of the incision for carpal tunnel surgery and is thus vulnerable to injury. The main "trunk" of this nerve is rarely injured in carpal tunnel surgery, but the nerve also has small terminal branches that lie just under the skin of the palm, and it may not be possible to make an incision in the palm without a chance of cutting small terminal nerve branches.

Surgeons are careful to protect any nerves encountered during surgery. If a nerve is large enough to be visible, the surgeon may avoid it or hold it to the side of the surgical field. In any case, surgeons always maintain an awareness of nerves' whereabouts. For very small microscopic nerves, surgeons try to avoid injury by not placing incisions where these small nerves are known to be located. Still, as mentioned, it may be impossible to make an incision in the palm of the hand without cutting small nerves, which can result in some scar sensitivity after carpal tunnel surgery. Again, the position and size of the scar that results from the endoscopic approach are reported to cause less scar sensitivity.

Another nerve subject to injury during carpal tunnel surgery is the recurrent motor branch of the median nerve, which provides the muscle power to the ball of the thumb. It branches from the main median nerve just at the end of the carpal tunnel, where it hooks around the transverse carpal ligament and enters the muscle. The origin of this nerve has been well studied, and there is some variation to its course, including one documented variation that puts this nerve in a very risky location. In this variation, the motor branch emerges from the ulnar side of the median nerve and crosses over the nerve to reach the ball of the thumb.

A patient with this anatomical pattern is at greater risk for injury to this important branch of the median nerve in any surgical approach; but the risk is perhaps greatest with the endoscopic technique. The sensory branches that come from the nerve and are destined for the fingers are also susceptible to injury if the endoscopic approach is used.

Finally, injury to the ulnar nerve and its sensory and motor branches is possible with all three techniques of carpal tunnel surgery because the ulnar nerve lies just outside the carpal tunnel. Again, however, such injuries are rare.

92 What happens if a nerve is cut during carpal tunnel surgery?

If a nerve is cut during surgery and the surgeon realizes this has happened, the nerve can be surgically repaired during the operation.

If the surgeon doesn't suspect that a nerve has been injured until after the surgery, repeat surgery may be needed to explore the problem and repair the laceration.

Sometimes patients report nerve symptoms that indicate possible injury to the median nerve during carpal tunnel surgery. The surgeon must evaluate the situation and may recommend repeat surgery to define the problem and, if necessary, repair any damage.

93 What types of treatment are available if carpal tunnel surgery doesn't work?

As mentioned earlier in this section, carpal tunnel surgery appears to give complete relief of symptoms in as many as 90 percent of patients. However, records on outpatient operations and repeat operations are not easily obtainable, and reports in medical journals estimate the number of failures significant enough to warrant further surgery at about 3 percent. Certainly the incidence of failures and recurrences is higher than that because many people who do not obtain complete relief from their symptoms decide against further surgery.

If you are continuing to experience symptoms, your doctor may try some nonsurgical treatments, including splinting, repeat injection, changes in activities on a trial basis, and even getting a new job if possible. Research suggests that repeat surgeries are less likely to help than the first one, so this should be considered only when you and your doctor have already tried everything else and there seems to be some chance that another surgery might help.

Several variations on the operative procedure can be used for repeat carpal tunnel surgery. The endoscopic technique should not be used because your surgeon should be able to observe and carefully inspect the median nerve during the operation. For the same reason, I would not recommend using the small-incision technique for repeat surgery.

Your surgeon might perform a repeat simple release, which I usually recommend. Or he could also release the carpal tunnel and then shift some tissue over or around the median nerve as a kind of padding to separate it from the scar. Surgeons use various types of tissue, including neighboring fat, muscle, or a combination of these, for this purpose, but we have not yet had enough experience with these procedures to know if they help.

Unfortunately, the complete cure rate for repeat carpal tunnel surgery is probably in the range of only 25 to 30 percent, and the percentage of patients who experience absolutely no benefit from repeat surgery is also 25 to 30 percent.

PART NINE

Taking Charge: Carpal Tunnel Syndrome Prevention and Self-Care

Introduction

When people become medical patients, they typically find themselves relieved of some of life's day-to-day responsibilities. They have permission to let others make decisions for them, and they're excused from taking part in some of the usual activities that are part of human existence.

This passive posture creates a special place for patients in our society, and, although it can be helpful in the face of life-threatening conditions or serious accidents, unfortunately, this social dynamic works against individuals with nerve compression. In my professional experience, I've noticed that people are happiest when they are actively engaged in life, when they are making good decisions about themselves, when they are planning for the future, and when they are pursuing their interests.

I have found that patients with nerve compression usually feel better and *are* better if they can take an active role in their medical management and in their lives. A large and growing body of recent medical evidence shows us that patients do better if they can participate in the decision making about their medical conditions. If you actively do everything you can to improve your health, and if you participate with your doctor in planning your care, you'll be more satisfied with your state of health even if you don't recover completely.

If you work at a job that you believe puts you at risk for carpal tunnel syndrome, or if you have numbness in your hands already, the exercises in the Appendix offer your best opportunity to prevent carpal tunnel syndrome from occurring. Research into the effectiveness of these exercises, developed at the Orthopedic and Reconstructive Research Foundation in Oklahoma City, has shown that they actually reduce pressure in the carpal tunnel. Performing them is a great opportunity for you to be proactive about your carpal tunnel health.

If you are experiencing new symptoms, if you are having trouble sleeping, if your hands are making you uncomfortable, definitely check with a doctor. But instead of asking, "What are you going to do to make my hands better?" ask, "What can you suggest that I might do to help myself get better?"

94 Can I do anything on a day-to-day basis to help relieve my symptoms?

Most of us can improve our overall health by paying more attention to our posture while sitting, standing, walking, and working.

With regard to upper limb problems generally, heavy purses, briefcases, and suitcases pull on the arm and can stretch the nerves in your neck, causing pain. Even if you don't have carpal tunnel syndrome, you may have noticed that you get numbness in the hand when you carry a heavy suitcase through an airport. This is a message from your brachial plexus, telling you that it is being stretched or compressed. Listen to your body and pay attention to what it is telling you.

Stretching and light strength training are valuable for most people. Improving your overall fitness may help to alleviate nerve symptoms as well as many other conditions, but see your doctor for a checkup before you embark on a fitness program.

95 Are there any exercises that can prevent or heal carpal tunnel syndrome?

H. Seradge, M.D., at the Orthopedic and Reconstructive Research Foundation in Oklahoma City, has devised a series of brief exercises that almost anyone can use to try to reduce pressure in the carpal tunnel.

These exercises are described in the Appendix. I recommend doing them before starting work or engaging in any other daily activity that may flex or extend the wrist for a prolonged period, and also after you finish the activity. They take only a few minutes to perform, but they may save you much suffering.

One note of caution: These exercises shouldn't cause you any pain. If they do, you should check with your doctor.

96 Is the Internet a reliable source of information about carpal tunnel syndrome and its treatment?

Although I believe that the Internet offers a great deal of useful information about carpal tunnel syndrome, I also think that you should take what you read with a grain of salt. Unlike the information in medical journals, anyone can put just about anything he likes on the Internet. There are few standards or "truth filters" for evaluating information before it reaches you on your computer.

Still, dozens of credible Web sites sponsored by medical organizations and medical centers offer legitimate, up-to-date, and valid information about medical conditions and medical care. A number of these sites are listed in the Resources section.

It's becoming increasingly common for people, including surgeons, to put information on the Internet as a form of advertising. This is definitely the case for carpal tunnel syndrome. Whether a site recommends surgery, splinting, or yoga, avoid blindly accepting recommendations that you find on the Internet. Read as much as you can, learn as much as you can, surf until your fingers get calluses, but remember that you and your doctor know what's best for your hands.

I do not recommend buying products for treatment of carpal tunnel syndrome from Internet sites. Numerous sites offer magnets, splints, how-to books, and other products and treatments, but you have no way of knowing how legitimate these businesses are, and charlatans can have very professional Web sites. You will have to pay shipping on everything you order, and you may find it difficult or impossible to get your money back if you aren't satisfied. For example, you should try on a splint to make sure it's comfortable before you pay for it. You won't be able to do that if you order online.

97 Can I decrease my chances of developing carpal tunnel syndrome if I use an ergonomic keyboard and chair?

My general rule is that you should try a chair or a keyboard for a period of time before you buy it. A number of ergonomic keyboards are available that change the position of the hand for typing. These may be split into two sections that slant outward. I don't know of any research that shows that these work, but the idea of using the hands in a slightly less palm-down position, letting the elbows hang straight down from the shoulders, and keeping the wrists in a straight line with the forearm rather than allowing them to ulnar-deviate (slant outward in the direction of the ulna) seems to make sense. I can only tell you to try before you buy.

Your chair is very important for your comfort. Pay attention to the position of your back and shoulders when keyboarding. Your feet should be in front of you on the floor and your knees and hips should form a right angle. Your back should be straight and your arms comfortable. Your wrists should be straight, not bending up or down. You might want to consider sitting in a higher chair so that you don't shrug your shoulders. Check out all these features before you buy a new chair or keyboard.

98 Until we know more about how work activities may affect carpal tunnel syndrome, how can I best take care of myself?

If you have a job that involves using a keyboard every day, but you don't have symptoms of carpal tunnel syndrome, you can guard against developing it by watching your posture and making sure that you keep your wrists straight when you are keyboarding.

The jury is still out regarding whether the various types of computer mice or pointing devices contribute to RSI conditions. I take a cautious stance and recommend that you avoid wearing watches and bracelets that might put pressure on the inner surface of the wrist when you rest it on any surface, including when you are working at a keyboard. It's possible that pressure on the wrist can push on the transverse carpal ligament and increase pressure within the carpal tunnel. Similarly, I advise against letting the wrist actually rest on any of the cushions or pads that are now being marketed. These pads on mouse pads and keyboards may help keep you from excessively flexing or extending your wrists, but I don't believe that the cushioning itself has any benefit. In fact, if you stop to notice, you'll see that the cushion may actually push on the carpal tunnel. Also, be sure to take frequent breaks and to use the exercises described in the Appendix.

If you're already having hand symptoms, try a splint at night for a month. If you don't get relief, see your family doctor or a hand surgeon.

Finally, no matter what your symptoms or condition, avoid dwelling excessively on blaming your workplace. You'll be much better off physically and emotionally if you take responsibility for changing what you can by being proactive about your health care and enjoying your life.

99 Are there any links between carpal tunnel syndrome and certain sports?

A number of sports activities have been linked with carpal tunnel syndrome. This isn't surprising, because the condition can be caused by certain postures of the hand and wrist, and some sports require specific positions of the wrists and strong gripping for prolonged periods of time.

Some sports that have been noted by enthusiasts and athletes to cause numbness of the hands include rock climbing, wheelchair basketball, weight lifting, windsurfing, and race-car driving. I am sure there are others. The common features of these sports that may be related to carpal tunnel syndrome are the hand posture and the strong gripping required.

Wheelchair athletes use their hands to propel themselves in their chairs. This may require extension or flexion of the wrist in combination with gripping. Weight lifters have been shown to develop nerve compression that is related to the length of time they have been engaged in the sport. These athletes put incredible strain on their muscles and joints. Also, when weight lifting is used as a method of bodybuilding, the athlete may have a very low body-fat content. The major nerves tend to be padded by fat, and I've noted a number of cases of cubital tunnel syndrome, or compression of the ulnar nerve at the elbow (see Part Two) among friends of mine who are weight lifters and body builders. I believe the loss of body fat leaves the ulnar nerve susceptible to irritation behind the elbow.

I've been told that windsurfing enthusiasts can develop numbness in the hands because the sport requires that riders hold a boom to control the sail. Experienced windsurfers use a harness to help reduce fatigue, and narrow booms are available that may reduce hand numbness, but I have no personal experience with the sport or these suggestions.

Rock climbers also report specific hand problems, including numbness. In addition, they can suffer from attenuation of the pulleys that hold the tendons tight to the fingers. Experienced climbers tape their fingers to avoid this problem.

If you are an athlete who has developed numbness in the hands, you should have a thorough medical checkup, primarily to make sure that a neck problem is not causing the numbness. If your doctor believes that carpal tunnel syndrome is the source of your symptoms, I recommend that you try night splinting (see Part Five) and the decompression exercises described in the Appendix.

100 Can alternative medicine treatments help carpal tunnel syndrome?

"Alternative medicine" refers to medical approaches and treatments that lie outside the mainstream of Western medicine as we define it today. Interest in alternative medicine and in blending alternative and mainstream medicine has exploded in the United States, and both the federal government and many universities are supporting research into alternative medicine.

A number of alternative therapies claim to be helpful in treating carpal tunnel syndrome. These include yoga, therapeutic massage, myofascial work, light therapy, and magnet therapy.

I find it hard to believe that these and other alternative therapies can reduce the pressure on the median nerve, so I doubt that they can help to cure true, progressive carpal tunnel syndrome. For example, I've noticed much recent interest in the use of magnets, which are placed against the body to relieve various symptoms, especially pain. Nothing in my Western medical training helps me to understand why placing a magnet close to the skin over the carpal tunnel would have any effect on the pressure affecting the median nerve, so I don't believe that magnets are of any value in treating carpal tunnel syndrome.

It's possible that some of these alternative treatments can help carpal tunnel syndrome patients by promoting feelings of well-being or through other means. It may be that some of the movements and manipulations involved in massage, stretching, yoga, and other alternative therapies have the indirect effect of decreasing pressure on the median nerve, but this is a matter for future research.

If a patient is interested in exploring an alternative treatment that I know will cause no further physical damage or harm and it isn't too expensive, I say, "Go ahead." By no means do we know all there is to know about carpal tunnel syndrome and how to treat it, and it's quite possible that some forms of alternative treatment may offer true benefits to patients. Perhaps some of these therapies will be proved effective and will soon become part of mainstream medical practice.

101 *What should I look for when considering alternative treatments for carpal tunnel syndrome?*

As in my comments about Internet information and products, my basic advice is, "Let the buyer beware." I wouldn't recommend spending a lot of money on unproven treatment methods.

Many of these treatments are heavily promoted by entrepreneurs on the Internet and elsewhere, and are quite costly. I advise caution in this area, especially if the product or treatment is expensive.

If you want to be active in treating your carpal tunnel syndrome on your own, your best and most affordable self-treatment is to buy a good wrist splint, wear it at night for a month, and see if it relieves your symptoms. Of course, general lifestyle improvement can help, too.

Some Closing Thoughts

Our research has shown that nerve symptoms are very common throughout the population. It's likely that you or a family member or friend has experienced numbness in the hands at some point in the past two weeks. It may have come from resting on your elbow, from sleeping in an awkward position, or from some other activity, but the symptom is common.

Our minds are always actively surveying our bodies for messages—the temperature, painful areas, grumbling in the stomach, and so on. We react to sensations by constantly interacting with our environment. We shift our weight on our chairs, we uncross one leg and cross the other, we scratch our heads or behind our ears. We're engaged in a constant subconscious gathering of information about the status of our bodies. If we have a symptom and then read about it, our minds will become more sensitized to it; from then on, we'll be scanning for that specific symptom.

So, if we read that numbness in our hands may be a sign of injury from using a computer keyboard or a computer mouse, this will register deep in our consciousness, and our brains will start looking for the occasional symptom of numbness. When it occurs, the brain, instead of simply responding by causing an automatic adjustment in our position, brings it to the level of consciousness. We become aware of the numbness and begin actively keeping watch for it. We notice the scattered instances of numbness that occur daily. We register the development of the symptom, and the symptom becomes amplified. Finally, it reaches the threshold where we perceive it as troublesome.

In the meantime, because we're curious about our problem, we begin reading about it. Newspaper stories, magazine articles, and books such as this one provide descriptions or templates for the possible disease process that we think we may have. Our symptoms become more focused, and we become more focused on our symptoms. We note those that fit the template, and we downplay those that we aren't experiencing, just as all medical students become convinced that they're riddled with one disease after another as they proceed through the curriculum. Finally, we reach a certain threshold where we decide to see a doctor, and we become patients.

My thoughts about health templates have been strongly influenced by Edward Shorter's writings on the changes in definitions of medical conditions on the part of both doctors and patients in history.

When the median nerve is mildly and intermittently compressed, as it is in many people, we may consider it a pathological condition, or just a symptom of life. However, at this early and mild stage of nerve symptoms, many types of intervention can have a positive effect. Some of these treatments need not even have any physiological effect on the nerve itself, because treatment can include behaviors, courses of action, or mental frameworks that change or influence how we survey our symptoms, how we interpret them, and the degree to which they will trouble us. Yoga, exercise, getting a hobby, therapeutic touch, light therapy, and many other interventions can change how you perceive symptoms and perhaps keep you from becoming a patient. Or, if you're already a patient, seemingly unconventional treatments may cure your problem. These ideas may not fit into orthodox medical thinking about health and disease, but I, like many of my colleagues, have seen their success in my practice.

Suppose that the nerve is compressed significantly. At this stage you'll begin developing symptoms that disturb your sleep and interfere with the use of your hand. If you don't receive treatment, the symptoms will worsen because you've reached a stage of compression that requires some form of mechanical intervention to relieve the pressure on the nerve. Trying nonsurgical treatments may help, and they'll also give you a chance to get to know your doctor and for your doctor to get to know you. Your symptoms may improve to a degree that you both decide you don't need surgery.

If it appears that surgery is the best course of action, however, learn as much as you want to about your problem. If you're going to make a wise decision, you should have some idea of what is likely to happen if you don't have surgery, what may occur if you try alternative treatments, and what may result if you have surgery.

Some surgeons are against "teaching" patients too much about their condition. Maybe the prospect of demystifying medical thinking threatens some doctors, who feel that their authority will be questioned. I suggest that you learn as much as you desire about your body and what is happening with it, that you ask your doctor as many questions as you wish to, and that you take an active, educated part in deciding to do what's best for you and your hand.

You may have a package of disease; for example, arthritis of the wrist, but your doctor will recommend treatment based not so much on the mere presence of the disease but on how much the symptoms bother you. In hand surgery today, we're moving away from considering patients as being in a state of "health" or "disease" and instead are evaluating "symptom severity" and "functional limitations," which are conditions that just may be a part of life.

You may have carpal tunnel syndrome, but you may also be able to control the symptoms by night splinting, modifying some of your activities, taking things a bit easier, and so forth. We must change our model from one of eradicating disease to symptom and functional improvement. This is our goal for most problems of the upper limb, including carpal tunnel syndrome.

If this book answers some of your questions and helps you in your treatment and recovery, it will have achieved its purpose.

Appendix

H. Seradge, M.D., at the Orthopedic and Reconstructive Research Foundation in Oklahoma City, has devised a series of brief exercises that almost anyone can use to try to reduce pressure in the carpal tunnel. You should do them before starting work or engaging in any other daily activity that may flex or extend the wrist for a prolonged period, and also after you finish the activity.

Carpal Tunnel Decompression Exercises

1. Extend your arms forward straight in front of you, palms facing downward, and extend both wrists and fingers acutely, as if you were doing a handstand or a pushup. In other words, keeping your fingers straight, lift the back of your hand (the hairy side) toward your forearm. Hold for a count of five.
2. Still holding your arms in front of you, straighten your wrists, making each forearm and wrist a straight line, and relax the fingers for a count of five.

3. Keep your arms straight out in front of you and make a tight fist with both hands. Bend your wrists, flexing them downward toward the inner (hairless) part of the forearm while holding the fist. Hold for a count of five.

4. Still holding your arms in front of you, straighten your wrists, making each forearm and wrist a straight line, and relax the fingers for a count of five.

5. Repeat these two exercises ten times, then let your arms hang, loose and relaxed, at your sides for several seconds.

6. Shake out your hands in a loose, relaxed manner for a few seconds.

These exercises are very simple and will cost you only a few minutes of time, and they may save you much suffering by reducing pressure in the carpal tunnel and by either preventing a problem or improving your chances for nonsurgical relief of your symptoms. If you have a suspected high-risk job, you should definitely take the time to do these exercises, as should anyone who is experiencing numbness of the hands.

Caution: These exercises should not cause you any pain. If they do, you should check with your doctor.

Glossary

anatomy The study of the structure of living things.

arthritis Inflammation of the joint. Causes pain, swelling, heat, and limitation of function of a joint.

axillary block anesthesia A technique in which local anesthetic medication is injected around the brachial plexus to block the major nerves to the arm and hand.

axon A long extension of a nerve cell that transmits electrical signals.

basal joint arthritis A common location for arthritis of the hand; occurs at the joint at the base of the thumb.

brachial plexus A plexus or comingling of nerves in the neck, under the collarbone, and in the upper arm. The nerves sort themselves into three large nerves that innervate the arm and hand.

brachial plexus block anesthesia Anesthesia technique using local anesthetic medication injected in the area of the brachial plexus.

carpal tunnel A tunnel at the wrist containing tendons and the median nerve.

carpal tunnel syndrome A medical condition consisting of a constellation of symptoms, primarily numbness, caused by compression of the median nerve in the carpal tunnel.

cautery An electrical device that creates a current and coagulates small blood vessels. It is used in surgery to stop small blood vessels from bleeding.

cervical spine The spine from the skull to the upper chest, in the area of the neck.

cholecystectomy Removal of the gallbladder.

clinical A term used to describe something as "at the bedside." It can be employed to describe a test or some type of treatment; for example, "That is a useful clinical test for carpal tunnel syndrome."

common palmar digital nerve Nerve from which the smaller nerves that transmit sensation from the adjacent sides of the fingers originate.

complications A negative event after illness, testing, or treatment.

computed tomography (CT) A linkage between x-rays and computers that provides clear pictures of parts of the body.

cubital tunnel syndrome A constellation of symptoms caused by compression of the ulnar nerve behind the elbow.

cumulative trauma disease (CTD) A disease process caused by the cumulative effect of repetitive trauma.

demographic data General information about a person such as age, gender, place of residence, education, occupation, and income level.

de Quervain's tenosynovitis An inflammation of the tendon sheath of the first dorsal compartment involving the tendons that assist in extension of the thumb. It causes pain with thumb extension, but does not cause numbness.

diagnosis (plural, diagnoses) The label or name of a patient's disease or illness. A differential diagnosis is a list of the most likely conditions that are considered as possible diagnoses.

digital nerve Nerve that provides the innervation of the digit. The common digital nerves are located in the palm and the proper digital nerves are located along the sides of each finger and the thumb.

distal radius One of the two long bones in the forearm. The other is the ulna. The radius is the forearm bone that is on the same side as the thumb. The distal part of the radius is the end near the wrist.

When you check your pulse at the wrist you are pushing the artery against the distal part of the radius. It is the most commonly fractured bone in the skeleton.

double crush syndrome A term used to refer to a nerve that is compressed in two locations.

electrodiagnostic testing A form of evaluation of the function of a peripheral nerve using small amounts of electrical current.

electromyogram (EMG) The measurement of electrical activity of the muscles. This is often done by inserting small needle electrodes into the muscle to measure its activity.

endoscopic An approach to surgery in which the surgeon looks into a body cavity using a fiber-optic scope. The technique is usually performed through small incisions and offers the possibility of rapid recovery after surgery.

endoscopic carpal tunnel release Carpal tunnel release performed with the help of a fiber-optic instrument.

epidemic A situation in which a disease occurs in greater than expected numbers.

extension Movement of bending the wrist toward the outer (hairy) surface of the arm.

fibrillation Small, ineffective contractions that give a muscle the appearance of wiggling like a bag of worms.

flexion Movement of bending the wrist toward the inner (hairless) surface of the arm.

flexor retinaculum Essentially the same structure as the transverse carpal ligament, but this term refers to its functional importance as a pulley for the flexor tendons.

flexor tendons Tendons that connect the flexor muscles in the forearm to the bones of the fingers, causing flexion of the fingers when the muscles contract.

foramina (singular, foramen) Openings in a bone. Often a nerve will go through a foramen to pass through a bone.

general anesthesia A type of anesthetic in which the patient is given medication to "put her to sleep," to induce an anesthetic state, and to prevent pain.

hamate bone One of the wrist bones that forms a wall on one side of the carpal tunnel.

hand therapist A person trained in rehabilitation techniques to improve and restore comfort and function to the hand after illness, injury, or surgery.

hypertrophic scar A scar that is thickened and firm. It will often be raised and red but stay within the boundaries of the original injury.

idiopathic Of unknown cause.

imaging Techniques to make a visual image of a part of the body.

impairment rating A measure of the permanent alteration of the hand after illness or injury. It will often form the basis for calculating a patient's financial settlement.

inflammation A standard reaction of the tissue to injury character- ized by heat, swelling, pain, redness, and loss of function.

innervates (innervation) Provides the nerve input. Innervation can be used to describe a territory of skin being innervated by a sensory nerve or a muscle being innervated by a motor nerve.

intervertebral disk A fibrous disk of tissue that cushions the verte- brae, or spinal bones. The spinal column is made of an alternating stack of disks and vertebral bones.

intravenous anesthesia An anesthetic technique in which local anes- thetic medication is injected into the venous system for distribution to the arm and hand. A double tourniquet is inflated on the arm to hold the medication in the arm.

laser Acronym for "light amplification by stimulated emission of radiation." This is a phenomenon that results when an energy supply causes atoms to increase and then decrease their orbital energy in a uniform amount. This results in light that is monochromatic and in phase.

latency The time for an impulse to travel a specific distance in a nerve. This is an important electrical measurement to determine if a patient has nerve compression.

local anesthesia A type of anesthesia in which the anesthetic agent is injected into the area of surgery, numbing the tissue. The medication blocks transmission of nerve impulses so there is no sensation.

lumbricals Small "wormlike" muscles in the palm of the hand that coordinate the activity of the fingers. The lumbricals originate on the flexor tendon and insert on the extensor tendon, creating a delicate balance between these two structures.

magnetic resonance imaging (MRI) A method to provide a picture of the internal structure of the body; produced by using a strong magnetic field.

maximal medical improvement (MMI) A term used to describe the patient's level of recovery. At MMI, the patient is not expected to improve dramatically, signifying that any impairment present will be permanent.

medial epicondyle The bump on the inside of the elbow. This is a process of the end of the humerus. The ulnar nerve lies just behind the medial epicondyle.

median nerve A large nerve that provides sensation to a portion of the hand and motor power to the muscles of the ball of the thumb.

medical history The information the doctor gathers by questioning the patient, or his or her family.

metacarpals Tubular-shaped bones of the back of the hand.

motor end plate The location where an axon makes contact with a muscle cell.

motor nerve A nerve that innervates a muscle.

multiple crush A term used to describe a nerve with multiple levels of nerve compression.

muscle atrophy (wasting) Shrinkage of the muscle.

myelin Insulating material surrounding axons.

nerve compression Pinching of a nerve. Often this is due to its passage through a confined space such as the carpal tunnel.

nerve conduction velocity The speed at which an electrical signal travels in a nerve. This is measured as part of electrodiagnostic testing of a nerve.

nerve tests A term used commonly to describe electrical testing of the nerves (see *electrodiagnostic testing*).

open carpal tunnel release The standard carpal tunnel procedure with an incision that allows inspection of the carpal tunnel and the median nerve.

orthotist A professional who fabricates orthotics or splints to protect, stabilize, or control the motion of a body part.

phalanges Tubular-shaped bones that make up the skeleton of the fingers and thumb.

Phalen's test A test performed in the physical examination described by Dr. George Phalen. The patient is asked to flex the wrists for one minute. In a positive test, the patient develops numbness in the median nerve distribution area during the test.

prevalence The proportion of people with a certain attribute.

prognosis The expected future outcome or result of a medical condition.

pronator syndrome A constellation of symptoms occurring as a result of compression of the median nerve under the pronator muscle. These symptoms are similar to those of carpal tunnel syndrome.

pronator teres muscle A muscle in the forearm that pronates the hand; that is, it turns the palm toward the floor.

provocative pressure test A test performed during the physical examination. The doctor pushes on the skin overlying the median nerve. A positive test results in symptoms of carpal tunnel syndrome.

provocative tests A type of physical examination test that provokes symptoms in patients with nerve compression. Phalen's test, the provocative pressure test, and Tinel's sign are examples of provocative tests.

radius One of the two large bones that form the skeleton of the forearm.

reflex sympathetic dystrophy (RSD) A rare, painful condition of the hand that can follow surgery or injury.

repetitive strain injury (RSI) Injury to the hand as a result of repetitive activity.

scaphoid bone A bone of the wrist that forms a wall of the carpal tunnel.

Schwann cells Cells that form the myelin insulation around axons.

sensory nerve A nerve that delivers sensory information to the spinal cord.

sign In the medical context, something the doctor notices or finds.

small-incision or mini-incision carpal tunnel release Release of the carpal tunnel through a small incision.

symptom Something the patient notices about himself or herself.

syndrome A constellation of symptoms that commonly occur together.

synovectomy Removal of the synovial tissue, which is the lining of a tendon or joint.

synovium (synovial tissue) The nutritional tissue lining joints and tendons.

thenar muscles Muscles that make up the ball of the thumb. They control a lot of the motion and coordination of the thumb.

thoracic outlet syndrome A constellation of symptoms caused by compression of the major nerves of the brachial plexus in the area of the collarbone and first rib.

Tinel's sign A physical examination sign for nerve injury. The nerve is tapped at the site of the suspected injury; a positive test results in an electrical sensation in the distribution area of the nerve.

tissue injury Damage to tissue that creates a patterned response of inflammation.

tomogram A form of x-ray in which the beam of radiation is repeated at different angles to provide a focused image of a part of the body.

traditional carpal tunnel release Standard open carpal tunnel release; allows the surgeon to visually inspect the carpal tunnel and median nerve.

transverse carpal ligament A strong, fibrous ligament that bridges the carpal arch, forming the roof of the carpal tunnel.

two-point discrimination A physical examination test in which the patient is asked to determine if one point or two points are touching the skin. This is a standard method to measure the sensibility of the skin. It is reduced in severe nerve compression.

ulna One of the two large bones that form the skeleton of the forearm.

ulnar nerve A large nerve of the forearm and hand that provides sensation to the small finger and half of the ring finger and motor power to most of the small muscles of the hand.

ultrasound A diagnostic technique using sound waves to image or measure some aspect of anatomy.

Resources

⊞

Books

The Carpal Tunnel Helpbook. Scott M. Fried, M.D., Perseus Publishing, Cambridge, Mass., 2001.

This handbook for self-healing by a hand surgeon contains two very informative and helpful chapters: "Nerve Problems in the Neck, Shoulders, Arms, and Hands" and "The Anatomy of Nerve Injury." The remaining chapters deal with a variety of nonsurgical treatments to improve nerve compression symptoms. Fried promotes a proactive approach to well-being and provides good information that will help you do the same.

Conquering Carpal Tunnel Syndrome and Other Repetitive Strain Injuries. Sharon J. Butler, New Harbinger Publications, Oakland, Calif., 1996.

This self-care program aims to help patients with repetitive strain injuries and carpal tunnel syndrome and to offer preventive guidance. Butler is not a surgeon, and I disagree with some of the information provided. For example, she assumes that carpal tunnel syndrome is a repetitive strain injury, a stance I question in the text of this book. Having said this, I believe that an exercise and stretching approach can be useful to prevent and treat carpal tunnel syndrome.

End Your Carpal Tunnel Pain Without Surgery. Kate Montgomery, Rutledge Hill Press, Nashville, Tenn., 1998.

This interesting book contains a lot of exercises for upper-extremity problems. It promotes the "Montgomery Method" developed by the author, a massage therapist and holistic health practitioner. The book is written from the perspective of a nonsurgeon, and some of the information is difficult to understand from a medical point of view. For example, the tests for "misalignment" on pages 22 and 23 do not seem to be based on anatomy or physiology, and I don't see any useful purpose to them. However, it's interesting to see a nonsurgeon's perspective on carpal tunnel syndrome, and it is possible that exercises and stretching, such as those shown in this book, could reduce pressure in the carpal tunnel and thus offer some benefit.

From Paralysis to Fatigue: A History of Psychosomatic Illness in the Modern Era. Edward Shorter, The Free Press, New York, 1992.

This fascinating book was written by a historian looking back at medical records while reflecting on the past to try to gain an understanding of medical conditions that have come and gone. Although written before the current debate over RSI in North America, this book lays out a possible mechanism for the genesis of this epidemic in tantalizing detail.

The Hand, Wrist, and Arm Sourcebook. Steven J. McCabe, M.D., and Stan Goldman, Ph.D., Lowell House, Los Angeles, Calif., 2000.

This sourcebook was written as an informative text to educate laypersons about the hand, its function, and its problems. Chapter 9 is devoted to carpal tunnel syndrome and Chapter 10 to other nerve compression problems. Chapter 17, "Understanding the Workers'

Compensation Maze," is particularly useful for people with work-related difficulties. It is an accessible, easy-to-read book for anyone interested in the marvels of the hand as well as its problems.

Light at the End of the Carpal Tunnel. Scott M. Fried, M.D., Healing Books, East Norriton, Pa., 1998.

Fried's first book is easy to read and informative. It relies heavily on anecdotal patient experiences to illustrate his points. Among the thirteen chapters are "Faith Healing Versus Faith in Healing," "Surgery—Who Should Have It? When and Why?," and "Biofeedback, Hypnosis, and Magic."

Stretching at Your Computer or Desk. Bob Anderson, Shelter Publications, Inc., Bolinas, Calif., 1997.

This short, easy-to-understand book offers stretching exercises for the entire body with dozens of helpful line drawings. These stretches may reduce pressure in the carpal tunnel. In any case, I believe overall stretching is important for general well-being.

Internet Web Sites

These Web sites give brief descriptions of carpal tunnel syndrome. If you search for "carpal tunnel syndrome," more than thirteen thousand Web sites appear. The sites I list here are generally accurate but tend to offer only brief, superficial descriptions of the syndrome.

http://orthoinfo.aaos.org

This Web site for the American Academy of Orthopedic Surgery has information about many common hand problems, including carpal tunnel syndrome, and other orthopedic conditions.

www.hand-surg.org

The American Society for Surgery of the Hand is one of two large professional associations for hand surgeons in the United States. This Web site offers patient information brochures, including some information on carpal tunnel syndrome.

www.carpal-tunnel.com/index.htm

This site, the "Carpal Tunnel Information Page," gives a brief description of carpal tunnel syndrome and its symptoms, causes, anatomy, prevention, diagnosis, and treatment, including a short discussion of surgery. It is also linked to a list of books at Amazon.com about carpal tunnel syndrome.

www.cdc.gov/niosh/ctsfs.html

This is the carpal tunnel syndrome information page for the National Institute for Occupational Safety and Health (NIOSH). This page has a brief description of carpal tunnel syndrome.

http://health.yahoo.com

This is a general health Web site (Yahoo Health) that offers accurate information on carpal tunnel syndrome and other compression neuropathies. It is concise and informative, and also has links to search for specific information.

http://webmd.com

This site, Web M.D., is a truly wonderful Web site that has extensive information about carpal tunnel syndrome. Pages of information cover every area of interest from alternative therapies to mini-incision carpal tunnel surgery. If you have time to browse, read, and think, I highly recommend this site.

www.drkoop.com

This site, sponsored by former U.S. Surgeon General C. Everett Koop, has several pages devoted to carpal tunnel syndrome, its causes, and its treatment. It contains some interesting reports of recent research. The information is brief but well written and informative.

www.intellihealth.com

This site is a medical Web site that contains a large volume of information. The general pages on carpal tunnel syndrome are comprehensive and appear accurate. I can't comment on the use of herbal remedies suggested on this site, but I think you'll find the information useful and educational.

Index

sutures, 86–87

synovectomy, 84

time for, 86

traditional open technique,
    82, 83–84, 99

transverse carpal ligament
    severed in, 18

when recommended, 71

carpal tunnel syndrome

acute, 24

causes, 2–3

as collection of symptoms, 3

defined, 2

determining severity of, 57–58

epidemiological evidence
    and, 32–33

history, 37–39

nerve compression in cervical
    spine and, 28

recurrent, 105

signs of, 3

as social and political issue, 2

wrist flexion and, 20

carrying heavy objects, 114

CAT scans, 63

cautery, 86

cervical arthritis, 26

cervical spine

compression of nerves in, 28

diagnosing nerve compres-
    sion in, 28–29

chairs, ergonomic, 116

children, 33, 86–87

clumsiness of hand, as a
    symptom, 4

collarbone, nerve compression
    in region of, 24–25, 26

common palmar digital nerve,
    10–11, 15, 16

complications of carpal tunnel
    surgery, 101–11

assessment of, 103

assigning blame for, 101–2

resolving difficulties, 102–3

from surgical injuries, 105

temporary relief, 105

from unrelated problems,
    104–5

compression of median nerve,
    1, 2. *See also* pressure in
    carpal tunnel

causes of, 1

congenital, 33

first recognition as cause of
    carpal tunnel syndrome, 38

nerve function and, 20–21

pressure in carpal tunnel
    syndrome and, 20

sleeping position and, 2, 22

compression of ulnar nerve, 7

cubital tunnel syndrome,
    24, 26

defined, 24

cumulative trauma disorder,
    49, 50, 51–52. *See also*
    repetitive strain injury